# THE
# MEMORY
# SOLUTION

## JULIAN WHITAKER, MD
### with PEGGY DACE

AVERY PUBLISHING GROUP

Garden City Park • New York

The therapeutic procedures in this book are based on the training, personal experiences, and research of the authors. As the sole purpose of this book is to educate, every effort has been made to provide the most complete, current, and accurate information as possible. It is not intended as a substitute for the medical advice of a trained health professional. The reader should consult his or her physician before adopting any of the suggestions presented in this book.

The publisher does not advocate the use of any particular health treatment, but believes the information provided in this book should be made available to the public. The authors and publisher are not responsible for any adverse effects or consequences resulting from the use of any of the suggestions or procedures described in this work.

Cover Designers: Jana Lewis
 and Phaedra Mastrocola
In-House Editor: Marie Caratozzolo
Typesetter: Richard Morrock
Printer: Paragon Press, Honesdale, PA

**Avery Publishing Group**
120 Old Broadway
Garden City Park, NY 11040
1–800–548–5757
www.averypublishing.com

**Library of Congress Cataloging-in-Publication Data**

Whitaker, Julian M.
    The memory solution: Dr. Julian Whitaker's 10-step program to optimize your memory and brain function / Julian Whitaker with Peggy Dace.
        p.   cm.
    Includes bibliographical references and index.
        ISBN   1–58333–023–2
1. Memory—Nutritional aspects.   2. Dietary supplements.   3. Nootropic agents.
4. Intellect—Nutritional aspects.   I. Dace, Peggy.   II. Title
    QP406.W47     1999
    612.8′2—dc21                                                                99–35379
                                                                                        CIP

Printed in the United States of America

10  9  8  7  6  5  4  3  2  1

# Contents

# Acknowledgments

We would like to acknowledge the invaluable assistance of researcher Kelley Griffin of the Whitaker Wellness Institute, editor Marie Caratozzolo for her fine skills, and Norman Goldfind of Avery Publishing Group for his help in putting this project together. Dr. Whitaker would like to thank his wife, Connie, and their eight children, Julian Jr., Tammy, Angelina, David, Shahana, Conrad, Louisa, and Max for their love and support. Peggy Dace would like to thank her husband, Bruce Boyd, and her sons, Bret, Brandon, and Ben, for their patience and love.

# Introduction

In May 1997, reigning world chess champion Garry Kasparov took on Deep Blue, a sophisticated supercomputer programmed to consider billions of chess positions, some 200 million moves per second. That the computer beat Kasparov is immaterial. That one man alone was a match for this engineering marvel, developed over decades with the input of dozens of programmers and chess grand masters, is testimony to the power of the human brain.

The complex calculations required to play a game like chess are just one function of your multifaceted brain. Within the three-pound mass encased in your skull originate the amazingly complex processes of reasoning and learning, memory, speech, and emotional expression. Furthermore, sensory perception and the automatic functions that keep you alive, such as breathing, thirst, hunger, and sleep, are all controlled by the brain.

Every moment of every day your brain performs incredible feats, some of which science and medicine are just beginning to understand. Yet we take for granted these miracles of everyday life—recognizing a face, recalling a phone number, solving a problem. Only when the ability to perform these routine tasks is lost or impaired do we consider the elegance and intricacy of the human brain.

The truth is that almost everybody experiences difficulties with memory and cognitive function at some time or another. It might be during a particularly stressful period, or after an injury or illness. But for most people, mental lapses and declines in cognitive function occur with advancing age, usually beginning in the fifth or sixth decade of life. Some might notice only occasional forgetfulness, while others may feel they've lost their mental edge—and the most severely afflicted, those with Alzheimer's disease, suffer irreversible, progressive brain degeneration. Yet even the most minor memory and cognitive slips are cause for concern. After all, memory and reasoning are what make us human—they are the essence of our beings.

I have been a practicing physician for over twenty-five years, specializing in the treatment of degenerative diseases such as heart disease, hypertension, diabetes, and arthritis. I didn't begin my practice with an expertise or interest in cognitive function. Thought and memory were the stuff of psychiatry. My interest in this field broadened, however, as I found that my patients were looking to optimize not only their physical health, but their mental function as well. It was their needs that led me to further my research into the workings of the brain, to understand why we experience age-related memory loss and how it can be prevented.

Early on I discovered the therapeutic power of vitamins, minerals, herbs, natural hormones, and "smart" drugs and nutrients. I also became aware of the irrational bias of conventional medicine, with its dependence on pharmaceutical drugs and surgical techniques, against these safe, effective therapies. I've pored over the scientific research that clearly establishes links between brain function and nutrition, exercise, stress, and other lifestyle factors. And I've examined hundreds of studies demonstrating how certain vitamins, herbs, amino acids, fats, hormones, and "smart" drugs and nutrients improve mental function. Most important, I've used these agents in my medical practice for over twenty years, and thousands of my patients have discovered firsthand that memory and cognitive function can be enhanced and restored.

In this book, I want to share with you the 10-step program these patients followed to regain and maintain their memory and sharpen their mental edge. Part One presents the mental changes you might expect with the passage of years, and lays to rest some of the myths about aging, memory, and intelligence. I'll then take you through a crash course on the physiology and workings of the human brain to familiarize you with concepts you'll meet again when we discuss the specific steps for improved brain function. We'll also look at factors that negatively affect the brain, and I'll tell you how you can protect yourself from these brain poisons.

In Part Two, I will present the details of my 10-step program to sharpen memory and mental edge. You will learn which foods promote optimal brain function, as well as the vitamins, minerals, herbs, and other nutritional supplements that nurture and support cognition. You'll see the important role that exercise (both physical and mental), stress reduction, and sleep play in keeping you mentally sharp. And I'll introduce you to the hormones and the "smart" drugs and nutrients that have been used successfully in gaining and maintaining one's mental edge. Part Two concludes with a chapter that ties it all together, summarizing how you can build your own brain-boosting program.

My wish for you, as it is for all of my patients, is optimal health, which encompasses body, mind, and spirit. By following my 10-step program, you will enjoy both a clearer, sharper mind and improved general health. May the recommendations in this book enhance your life, as they have so many others, and set you on the path to good health.

Best of health,
Julian Whitaker, MD

# PART ONE

# Memory, Intelligence, and the Brain

# CHAPTER 1

---

# Memory Loss Is Not Inevitable

*Hal, a fifty-six-year-old marketing manager, meets with and talks on the phone to dozens of people every day. Remembering names and faces, as well as tidbits about his clients, is crucial, and he has always prided himself on how well he does this. Lately, however, Hal feels he's slipping. He'll know the face, but can't immediately place the name. He'll start to ask about the family, but can't remember the wife's name. It's more of an occasional nuisance than a real problem, and cues in the conversation invariably jolt his memory. But in his highly competitive industry, Hal sometimes worries about losing his edge.*

Does Hal's situation sound familiar? Do you find yourself forgetting names, misplacing your eyeglasses or keys, losing your train of thought in the middle of a sentence, or (my favorite) walking into a room and suddenly not remembering why you're there? Let me assure you that you are experiencing nothing out of the ordinary. A name forgotten here, a misplaced item there—these are everyday occurrences that can happen to anyone, at any age. If you've raised children, you know that kids forget everything—chores, homework, where they put their shoes, you name it. Yet we don't worry about their memories.

However, once you've hit your forties or fifties, especially as you notice the more visible signs of aging such as graying hair and vision problems, you tend to become more alarmed by these ordinary mental lapses. Misplaced keys become a harbinger of senility, forgotten phone numbers a sign of early Alzheimer's disease. According to a recent survey, the major health fear of older Americans is not heart disease and cancer—our number one and number two killers. It's Alzheimer's disease. Pain, disability, medications, and hospitalizations we can handle. The idea of succumbing to memory loss—losing our "selves," in a sense—and becoming a burden to our families is much more frightening.

With all the press Alzheimer's disease is getting these days, it's no wonder we construct these gloom-and-doom scenarios. It almost seems inescapable, doesn't it? Well, it isn't. The stereotype of the dotty, forgetful senior citizen is a myth, nothing more. The truth is, most people glide into their golden years with great awareness and perspective. And many remain intellectually active well into their eighties and nineties. After winning two Nobel prizes, including the Nobel Peace Prize, Dr. Linus Pauling published his best-known work, *Vitamin C and the Common Cold*, at age sixty-nine. English poet Robert Browning died in 1889 at the age of seventy-seven, the day his last volume of poetry was published. George Bernard Shaw, the Irish playwright who was awarded the Nobel Prize for Literature in 1925, continued writing into his nineties. Spanish artist Pablo Picasso remained an innovative and creative force in the art world throughout his ninety-one years.

Of course, you have only to look around you to know that some people do, in fact, develop memory problems, and others suffer severe forms of dementia. On the surface, it may appear to be a crapshoot or a lottery draw—the lucky ones retain their faculties, while the unfortunates lose out. This couldn't be further from the truth. The message of this book is that memory loss and mental declines are neither random nor inevitable. And I'm going to show you how you can protect your brain, enhance your mental edge, and remain alert, focused, and intellectually productive throughout your life.

## MEMORY LOSS: DEBUNKING THE MYTHS

The natural, lifelong course of memory and mental function has been demonstrated clearly in data gathered over the past few decades from the Baltimore Longitudinal Study on Aging. This study, conducted by researchers at the Johns Hopkins Medical Center and funded by the National Institute on Aging, is the most ambitious research project to date on the mysteries of aging. Begun in 1958 and continuing into the next century, this study focuses on normal healthy individuals, the category into which the vast majority of you fall. This type of research is a breath of fresh air because, unlike most studies, it focuses on normal aging, not on Alzheimer's disease, heart disease, arthritis, or any other age-related illness. And it underscores a serious problem with the bulk of medical research.

We spend billions of dollars a year studying illness, comparing one pharmaceutical drug with another, exploring the pros and cons of various surgical interventions, and looking for the origins of disease. While this type of research is absolutely reasonable and valid, doesn't it make sense to direct at least a portion of our research dollars towards studying wellness? Rarely do studies address how to achieve optimal health through all the stages of our lives.

The Baltimore Longitudinal Study on Aging has provided some very surprising and encouraging findings on how we age. Among the most interesting is how our brains age. By following over 2,400 volunteers who return to Johns Hopkins every two years—some of them for over thirty years now—for two-and-a-half days of intensive medical testing, researchers have found that mental capacity is surprisingly stable as we age. Yes, there is some short-term memory loss and a slowdown in reaction time. But for the most part, in the absence of disease (such as Alzheimer's) or injury (stroke or trauma), cognitive function remains essentially intact throughout life. Vocabularies continue to increase. Reasoning skills flourish. Learning ability and intelligence do not decline.

A similarly designed study, the Seattle Longitudinal Study, began in 1956. Involving over 5,000 people, this study has found comparable results. Dr. K. Warner Schaie has spearheaded several investigations in this ongoing study on the lifelong course of mental and intellectual abilities, and found that many people live their entire lives without any noticeable declines in cognitive function.

## AGE-RELATED MEMORY IMPAIRMENT

Although the good news is that you can look forward to many years of normal brain functioning, our brains do gradually undergo changes as we age. Connections between brain cells or neurons disappear, and the brain literally shrinks in size. In addition, free-radical damage and other mechanisms of aging, which we will discuss in Chapter 3, take their toll. Levels of important brain chemicals called *neurotransmitters* decline, and circulation of blood, which delivers vital oxygen and nutrients to the brain, often becomes restricted.

In many people, memory and cognitive skills slip, a phenomenon known as *age-associated memory impairment*. This often begins in our forties and gets worse as we get older. A 1994 survey conducted by the Charles A. Dana Foundation found that 56 percent of respondents reported losing things frequently at age

## You May Be Sharper Than You Think

*Three women were discussing the travails of getting older. One said, "Sometimes I catch myself standing in front of the open refrigerator without a clue as to what I'm looking for."*

*The second woman chimed in, "Yes, every once in a while I find myself on the landing of the stairs and can't remember whether I was on my way up or on my way down."*

*The third one responded, "Well, I'm glad I don't have that problem—knock on wood." She rapped her knuckles on the table, then said, "That must be the door. I'll get it!"*

Unlike the third woman in this joke, which I picked up on the Internet, most people tend not to underestimate their mental declines but to overestimate them. They worry that they may be on the verge of senility, when all they are experiencing is normal age-related memory loss. Occasional memory lapses like those of the first two women in this joke are nothing out of the ordinary. The third one? Well, she needs to follow the 10-step program presented in this book!

forty-five, while 75 percent did so at the age of seventy-five. Forty-six percent of the forty-five-year-olds had trouble remembering names of familiar people; more than 50 percent had the same difficulties at seventy-five. At forty-five, 10 percent reported getting temporarily lost in familiar places; 20 percent did so at seventy-five.

Other areas in which age-related declines are noticed include all aspects of short-term recall, attention span, reaction time, tip-of-the-tongue memory (page 15), and multitasking—the ability to do more than one thing at a time. Unfortunately, these are such crucial functions, so important in both our careers and day-to-day living, that deficits can be at best a nuisance and at worst a liability.

## HOW WE REMEMBER

Before you get too concerned about declines in memory and mental function, let's take a quick look at how you remember things in the first place. Your brain has two basic storage systems for memory: working memory (also called short-term memory) and long-term memory. Your *working memory* is the entrance point for anything you see, hear, taste, smell, or touch, but this information doesn't necessarily linger or become a permanent memory. Working memory is limited by capacity—it holds roughly six or seven "chunks," or bits, of information and lasts anywhere from a few seconds to a few hours. Your working memory is in gear when you get a phone number from an operator, dial it, and then promptly forget it. It's what allows you to notice your environment, yet not clutter your memory with unnecessary details.

However, if what you observe or experience is different enough or important enough, it passes from working memory to *long-term memory* for retrieval later. The observation of a double rainbow after a thunderstorm or the birthday of your new grandchild will probably make it from working memory to long-term memory—the first because it's a rare experience and the second because it's emotionally significant. But the fact is that most of what you see, hear, taste, touch, or even reflect upon doesn't make it past working memory. It is simply used as needed, from moment to moment, then discarded.

Long-term memory, as its name implies, is much more durable. How strong long-term memories are depends on several factors. Attention and repetition are the primary means by which memories become indelible. The more you think about something, study it, turn it over in your mind, the stronger the memory becomes. Another factor is emotion. Emotion locks in memory, and fear is an especially powerful key. This is likely an evolutionary survival tool. It takes only one frightening face-to-face encounter with a snake or other animal—or even a scary story about such a beast—to propel you out of harm's way during future encounters. Other emotions, both positive and negative, also fortify memory. And when we recall, often in vivid detail, these memories, their emotional underpinnings also surface. Most of us can remember where we were when President Kennedy was shot or when the Challenger space shuttle blew up, and perhaps we even feel a surge of emotion at the memory. The shock and sadness of these tragedies solidified the memories. And on a more positive note, who can forget their first love?

Olfactory or smell-related memory is often emotion laden and particularly strong and lasting. Most of us have emotional reactions to particular smells. As a doctor's son growing up in the 1950s, I had my share of penicillin shots. To this day when I smell rubbing alcohol my hip starts to ache. A whiff of Ben-Gay and I'm back in my high school locker room, suiting up for a football game. For some, the fragrance of a certain perfume may evoke a long-lost love. For others, the smell of cinnamon rolls or apple pie might transport them back to their mother's kitchen. What scents conjure up memories for you?

The best news about long-term memory is that it seems to have infinite storage capacity. There's no limit to how much you can remember—the information just has to get there in the first place. Now let's look at what causes us to forget.

## WHY WE FORGET

As you can see, even in those who are young and healthy, memory is extremely selective. We forget much more than we remember. It's meant to be that way. Learning and forgetting, replacing old behaviors and thought patterns with new, are what make us adaptable and different from lower animals with innate, fixed behaviors. Our brains are programmed to tune out most of the sensory information we encounter—and to forget most of what is registered. And even then, if they are not brought into our consciousness frequently, many memories fade. But beyond the general way our brains are wired to forget, there are other reasons our memories falter. Psychologist William Cone, Ph.D., breaks these reasons into four categories—stimuli and filtering errors, "helpful" forgetting, the "tip-of-the-tongue" phenomenon, and time and memory.

## "Chunking" Numbers for Better Recall

The average person can hold up to six or seven bits of information in his or her working memory at one time. This is the reason telephone numbers are seven digits long. So how is it then, that most people are able to remember their nine-digit social security numbers? The answer lies in "chunking" or placing the numbers in smaller groups of two, three, or four. Grouping numbers increases your capacity to remember them. To illustrate this, try the following:

*Read the following string of numbers aloud, cover them, then try to repeat them in order.*

4 8 2 5 6 2 8 1 9

*Now, break the numbers into smaller groups, and try it again.*

4 8 2    5 6 2    8 1 9

If you're like most people, you found it easier to recall the numbers that are grouped. Typically, it is easier to remember three or four "chunks" of numbers, rather than a string of consecutive ones.

## Stimuli and Filtering Errors

Too many or too few stimuli negatively affect memory. There must be adequate stimulation from the senses to trigger the nervous system, but too many incoming messages can be overwhelming. The inability to read, study, or otherwise concentrate in the presence of a blaring TV and multiple background conversations is an example of overstimulation. (I've always been amazed at how teenagers manage to study with high-decibel rock-and-roll music in the background.) On the other hand, a housebound elderly person with a limited social network may have memory deficits as a result of understimulation. In a similar vein, if hearing, eyesight, or sense of smell and taste diminish or fail, sensory input is also limited and memory may suffer from lack of stimulation.

As I mentioned earlier, much of what we take in through our senses just doesn't merit remembering. Our long-term memories don't store all the details of everyday life, which explains why it's hard to remember what you had for lunch the day before yesterday. It's not that you forgot—this unessential information just never made it out of your working memory into long-term storage. This is known as *filtering*. Under certain circumstances, however, such as stress and worry, filters break down.

Notice how when you're under stress everything bothers you? You're edgy and ultrasensitive, and your thinking is muddled. This is primarily a filter/stimulus overload problem, compounded by exposure to stress hormones that impair the area of the brain where memories are processed. Likewise, when you're worried, you tend to focus on unfinished business, on what you should or shouldn't do, and this fills your consciousness, filtering out other perhaps more important thoughts. Information overload dampens memory in a similar way. You can process only so much information at once. Remember, your working memory can handle only six or seven information chunks, and when that limit is exceeded, information processing simply shuts down. We'll further discuss the impact stress has on your memory and how you can minimize its negative effects in Step 7 of my 10-step program in Part Two.

## "Helpful" Forgetting

Sometimes unpleasant memories are best forgotten. This may be accomplished consciously or unconsciously. For example, you may forget a dental appointment because you really don't want to go. Or you may intentionally refuse to think of something embarrassing or hurtful. The emotions associated with these thoughts are not forgotten and may be behind some of the phobias and fears people experience.

## The "Tip-of-the-Tongue" Phenomenon

A common type of memory failure that we've all experienced is being unable to recall something that you just *know* you know. "It's on the tip of my tongue." "I can see the face but can't recall the name." Although scientists have studied this phenomenon for years, we really don't understand much about it. Anyway, in most cases, the forgotten name or fact comes to you eventually, often when you're least expecting it.

Another aspect of this phenomenon is the feeling that there's something you need to do or think about, but it completely slips your mind. For example, you walk into a room and can't remember why you're there. In these cases, a cue from the environment or backtracking in your mind usually brings back the memory.

## Time and Memory

How often you recall something affects the durability of the memory. I've helped my children practice memorizing the states and their capitals, and although I myself once knew them all, I've forgotten a fair number of them. Why? Because I haven't needed to know this information for many years. You may no longer remember the phone number or address of a house you lived in years ago because you no longer need to know it.

As time goes by, memory becomes distorted. Although it may have rained every day during the fishing trip you took with your son years ago, and no one got more than a nibble, that trip—perhaps because of the emotional connection you made with your son—is remembered as the paragon of fishing trips. The weather was great, and the fish you caught, monsters all of them!

## DOES ALL MEMORY LOSS LEAD TO ALZHEIMER'S DISEASE?

Unfortunately, not everyone eases gracefully into his or her later years with perfect—or even acceptably average—memory and mental function. Most of you probably know someone, perhaps even a family member, who has Alzheimer's disease or another type of dementia. Alzheimer's disease affects 4 million Americans, and its incidence is expected to quadruple as the baby boomer generation ages.

Contrary to popular belief, Alzheimer's disease is not synonymous with dementia. Nor does everyone with age-associated memory impairment (which is common after age forty-five and involves minor disturbances in short-term recall, attention span, and reaction time) develop Alzheimer's disease. Although the symptoms of age-associated memory impairment are similar to the symptoms of early Alzheimer's, the two conditions are completely separate. Most people with mild to moderate memory lapses will not develop Alzheimer's disease.

Furthermore, not all cases of serious cognitive dysfunction or dementia are Alzheimer's disease. Many of them—even some erroneously diagnosed as Alzheimer's—are reversible. Best of all, as discussed in Chapter 3, many of the causes of dementia and cognitive dysfunction can actually be prevented.

## CAN I REALLY GET SMARTER?

In any discussion of memory and mental function, the question of intelligence always comes up. Can we get smarter and improve our intelligence quotient (IQ), or is intelligence fixed throughout life?

Before we address this, let's answer this question: What is intelligence? Most of us would have a hard time defining it, although we know it when we see it. Many feel intelligence is dependent on education and degrees. Others believe it's what is

# Memory Cues

The following test exemplifies the "tip-of-the-tongue" phenomenon discussed on page 15. Here's what you do: While keeping the column on the right covered, quickly run down the list of states on the left and name their capitals. Do this rapidly. Now, uncover the right column, which contains the first initials of the capital cities, and go through the list again. The letter cues should help jog your memory. (Answers on page 18.)

| State | First Letter of Capital City |
|---|---|
| Arizona | P |
| California | S |
| Colorado | D |
| Connecticut | H |
| Florida | T |
| Idaho | B |
| Indiana | I |
| Kansas | T |
| Louisiana | B |
| Michigan | L |
| Montana | H |
| Nevada | C |
| New Mexico | S |
| New York | A |
| Ohio | C |
| Pennsylvania | H |
| Rhode Island | P |
| Texas | A |
| Utah | S |
| Virginia | R |

**CAPITAL CITIES OF THE STATES LISTED ON PAGE 17:**

*Arizona*—Phoenix

*California*—Sacramento

*Colorado*—Denver

*Connecticut*—Hartford

*Florida*—Tallahassee

*Idaho*—Boise

*Indiana*—Indianapolis

*Kansas*—Topeka

*Louisiana*—Baton Rouge

*Michigan*—Lansing

*Montana*—Helena

*Nevada*—Carson City

*New Mexico*—Sante Fe

*New York*—Albany

*Ohio*—Columbus

*Pennsylvania*—Harrisburg

*Rhode Island*—Providence

*Texas*—Austin

*Utah*—Salt Lake City

*Virginia*—Richmond

measured with standard IQ tests. Intelligence, according to *Webster's New World Dictionary*, is "the ability to learn or understand from experience; ability to acquire and retain knowledge; mental ability"; or "the ability to respond quickly and successfully to a new situation; use of the faculty of reason in solving problems, directing conduct, etc., effectively."

Nowhere in these definitions does intelligence refer strictly to book learning and IQ tests. True, these do require and measure a certain type of intelligence, but they ignore other, equally important expressions of intelligence. In his book *Frames of Mind*, Harvard psychologist Howard Gardner, Ph.D., makes a case for the existence of seven types of intelligence:

- *Linguistic intelligence*—the ability to express ideas through speaking and/or writing. If you have a talent for writing, storytelling, public speaking, and debate, you have strong linguistic intelligence.

- *Logical/mathematical intelligence*—the ability to work with numbers and abstract reasoning. People with this type of intelligence are great problem solvers, able to do complex mental arithmetic and understand abstractions.

- *Spatial intelligence*—the capacity to perceive and visualize images and reproduce them spatially. People with spatial intelligence are the artists, architects, builders, and scientists of the world.

- *Musical intelligence*— skill in hearing and reproducing tone, rhythm, and pitch. If you have an ear for music, and singing or playing an instrument comes naturally to you, you shine in this type of intelligence.

- *Kinesthetic intelligence*—the ability to control movements of the body. Athletes, dancers, actors, and people with fine motor skills have kinesthetic intelligence.

- *Interpersonal intelligence*—the facility to interact with others. If you are a "people person," able to empathize, get along, work well with and motivate others, your interpersonal intelligence is keen.

- *Intrapersonal intelligence*—the capability to understand the inner self. People with this type of intelligence are tuned into their emotions and realize their own strengths and weaknesses.

With this broader view of intelligence in mind, I think you'll all agree without hesitation that yes, intelligence can be expanded throughout life—you can get smarter. Even the classic IQ definition of intelligence can be improved upon with the methods discussed in the 10-step program presented in Part Two.

## WE ALL HAVE UNIQUE LEARNING STYLES

In addition to having individualized expressions of intelligence, we also have unique learning and memory styles. There are four primary styles of learning—visual, verbal, auditory, and kinesthetic, and most of us are more proficient in one of these styles.

- *Visual learners* remember new information best when it is demonstrated or pictured. They best understand a scientific or mathematical concept by seeing it drawn out. They are the people who can, for example, watch someone whip up a gourmet dish, then reproduce it perfectly in their own kitchens.

## Emotional Intelligence

We all know people who are smart and successful in their line of work, but whose personal lives are a mess. And we know others who have a reputation for intelligence in a certain area, but who may not be able to find their way out of a paper bag. Although these people may excel in IQ, they may be sorely lacking in emotional quotient (EQ). In his book *Emotional Intelligence,* Daniel Goleman convincingly argues that the true indicator of a person's success in life is not rational but emotional intelligence—personal motivation, empathy, persistence, enthusiasm, self-discipline, and altruism. People with high EQs have meaningful relationships and strong family ties. They also succeed in their careers, not because they are the smartest kids on the block, but because of all the other qualities that success entails. And like other types of intelligence, emotional intelligence can be enhanced.

- *Verbal learners* retain most through reading, a skill highly prized in our schools. Many of our top students are verbal learners. They can learn how to use a computer, for example, simply by reading the manual.

- *Auditory learners* do best by hearing material presented aloud. These are the students who sit through lectures, never crack a book, and yet make good grades. They can hear something on TV or the radio and repeat it perfectly.

- *Kinesthetic learners* pick up things by doing—they're hands-on people. Take, for example, an athlete who cannot learn moves from a playbook, but has them down pat once he's walked through them.

What is your learning style? In which areas of intelligence do you excel? As a medical school graduate and physician, I've had to demonstrate a fair degree of linguistic and logical intelligence, and, as a recreational athlete, a share of kinesthetic intelligence. I tend to learn best by reading and listening. I've always had such admiration for people with high spatial intelligence, those who can build and create things with their hands. I am undeniably weak in that area!

As we discuss memory and how the brain works in the next chapter, and walk through the 10-step program in Part Two, I want you to focus on your unique intellectual gifts and learning style. Remember, we will be using the terms *intelligence, mental function,* and *cognitive function* (which encompass memory, language, and creativity) broadly to refer to all types of intelligence. But whatever you call them, all require a sharp memory and a well-functioning brain, which is what this book is all about.

# CHAPTER 2

# How Your Brain Works

*T*he brain has fascinated man since the dawn of mankind. Archeologists have found skulls dating back to the Stone Age that had holes bored into them—evidence of prehistoric cranial surgery. For much of human history, the predominant view was that the heart ruled the body. Among the first to challenge that view was Hippocrates, the Father of Medicine, who in the fifth century BC asserted, ". . . I am of the opinion that the brain exercises the greatest power in the man." In 300 BC, Greek physician and anatomist Herophilus made strides in understanding the physiology of the brain and nervous systems. About 100 years later, Galen, the physician to the Roman gladiators, reported on the effects of trauma to the brain. He was the first to note that certain areas of the brain are specialized to carry out specific functions. In the mid 1800s, French physician Dr. Paul Broca first identified the speech center of the brain after performing an autopsy on a man who had had severe speech difficulties. Over the next century, other functions—physical movement, the senses, learning, and emotions—were mapped to different areas of the brain.*

Since the late 1980s, we have witnessed great strides in imaging techniques and molecular biology, enabling us to understand more of the brain's secrets. Yet, despite these advances, the human brain remains an awe-inspiring, largely undiscovered frontier. As neurosurgeon Dr. Wilder Penfield, author of *The Mystery of the Mind*, aptly stated, "The workings of the mind will probably always be impossible to explain simply on the basis of electrical or chemical action in the brain and nervous system."

## THE ANATOMY AND PHYSIOLOGY OF THE BRAIN

I would like to take you on a brief guided tour of your brain. This is not intended to be an in-depth dissection of this complicated organ. I want only to familiarize you with the general concepts and terms we'll be referring to in my 10-step program for improving your memory and mental edge.

The physical mass of the brain is deceptively simple—three pounds of nerve cells, or neurons, in a supportive network of neuroglia, or glial cells, encased in the protective, bony cranium. This small mass is divided into four cavities, or ventricles, that are surrounded by and filled with cerebrospinal fluid that absorbs shock, maintains pressure inside the cranium, and transports important chemicals within the brain. As seen in Figure 2.1, the brain is composed of three major interconnected structures—the brain stem, the cerebellum, and the cerebrum. Each of these structures has different, but sometimes overlapping, functions.

### The Brain Stem

Located at the base of the brain atop the spinal cord, the *brain stem* is comprised of the *medulla* (or *medulla oblongata*), the *pons,* and the *midbrain.* The brain stem exits the skull and tapers into the spinal column; its job is to relay messages from the rest of the body to the cerebral cortex. The brain stem is sometimes called the "reptilian brain," as it is ancient in evolutionary terms and is similar to the simple brains of reptiles. The brain stem controls many of your most basic biological functions, such as heartbeat, blood pressure, and breathing.

Running through the brain stem is a structure called the *reticular formation,* which determines your state of alertness. The *reticular activating system* filters out much of the repetitive, familiar sensory input you are constantly bombarded with, but makes sure that strong or unusual impulses get your attention.

If other areas of your brain were damaged, but your brain

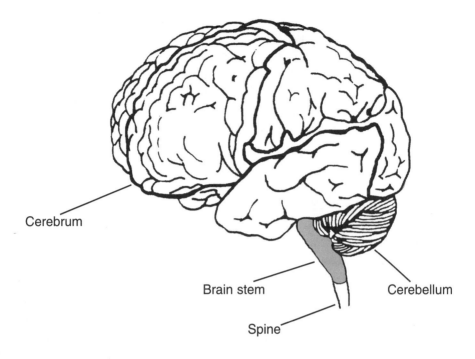

**Figure 2.1. The Brain**

stem was left intact, that most basic, instinctive part of your brain would keep you alive—comatose and vegetative, perhaps, but alive. However, damage to the brain stem often results in immediate death.

## The Cerebellum

The cerebellum ("little brain") lies over the medulla and the pons. It controls movement, coordination, muscle tone, and equilibrium. The reason the movements of infants are largely uncontrolled is because their cerebellums are not yet developed. Dancers and athletes, on the other hand, who display excellent coordination and a broad repertoire of controlled movements, have well-developed cerebellums. In addition, they display another function of the cerebellum, *memory of movement.*

You've experienced memory of movement yourself. You probably learned to ride a bicycle as a child, and, if you recall, mastering it wasn't easy. However, even if you haven't been on a bike in thirty years, within seconds of hopping on one, you'll be off and riding. You don't have to relearn how to ride. Your cerebellum has stored the specific physical maneuvers required to ride a bike as movement memory. Obviously, disease or injury to the cerebellum results in muscle and coordination problems, such as jerky, disjointed movements.

## The Cerebrum

Nobel laureate Dr. Roger Sperry described the cerebrum as "the crowning achievement of some five hundred million years of evolution." It occupies most of the cranium, weighs about two pounds, and is divided into two domes or hemispheres, which are connected by a cord-like band of nerve fibers called the *corpus callosum*. It looks a little like a walnut—two halves joined in the middle with a convoluted, wrinkled surface, protected by a hard outer shell. The cerebrum is sometimes called the "mammalian brain" because, in evolutionary terms, it is the youngest area of the brain and is unique to mammals. Snakes and lizards do not have a cerebrum; cats and dogs do, which explains why these mammals display more "human" traits of intelligence and affection and make better pets than reptiles.

The gray matter covering the cerebrum is called the *cerebral cortex* or *neocortex*. The cerebral cortex is thin, averaging $1/8$ to $1/10$ of an inch in thickness, but its fissures and grooves give it a much larger surface area. It is this thin layer of tissue that distinguishes the human brain from that of other animals, since it is responsible for the essence of humanity—thinking, learning, and remembering. Information from the five senses is received in an area of the cerebrum called the *sensory cortex*, and signals for action are relayed to the body from the *motor cortex*, both of which bisect the cerebral cortex in parallel bands.

The cerebrum is separated into right and left hemispheres. And it is further divided into four individual lobes.

### The Right and Left Hemispheres

You've probably heard the terms "left-brained" or "right-brain activity." This refers to the fact that while the two hemispheres of the cerebrum are more or less symmetrical (actually, the left hemisphere is larger in the areas devoted to language), their functions differ. The left hemisphere controls the right side of the body and orchestrates analytical, logical processes. The faculty for language, mathematical abilities, and analytic thought are more dominant in the left hemisphere. Abstract thought, emotions, appreciation of music and art, and spatial visualization are generally the domain of the right hemisphere, which controls the left side of the body. The left side of the brain is somewhat better developed in men than in women, which may explain why, generally speaking, men tend to do better in mechanics, engineering, and other analytic functions.

Along this same line, the corpus callosum, which connects the right and left hemispheres, is generally thicker in women than in men, allowing for more communication between the two hemispheres. It has been speculated that a thicker corpus callosum facilitates the interplay of emotion and logic, and that this is the basis of "female intuition."

This specialization and compartmentalization of the brain accounts for the predictable deficits that result from injury to certain areas of the brain. It explains why a person who has had a stroke or trauma localized to the frontal lobe may be able to understand spoken language, but be unable to express himself verbally. These deficits are sometimes peculiar. A famous case from the annals of neurology is that of H.M., whose hippocampus was surgically destroyed to successfully treat a long history of convulsions and seizures. H.M. retained his perceptual abilities, and his IQ even increased, but he was unable to remember anything for more than a few hours—short-term memories simply could not be moved into long-term storage. He lived in a state of constant disorientation, describing it like this: "Every day is alone in itself—whatever enjoyment I've had and whatever sorrow I've had."

### The Four Lobes of the Cerebral Hemispheres

Each half or hemisphere of the cerebrum is separated into four interconnected lobes, as seen in Figure 2.2. While each lobe specializes in certain functions, there is much shared work among the various areas. The *frontal lobes,* which comprise half of each hemisphere, are involved in deliberation, judgment, persistence, problem solving, and the regulation of action. Because of frontal lobe activity, we are able not only to focus our attention and learn, but also to restrain our impulses and act in a socially accepted manner. It has been suggested that attention deficit disorder, characterized by lack of focus and inability to control behavior, may originate in the frontal lobes. A part of the brain that functions in the production of speech, known as *Broca's area,* is also located in the frontal cortex.

Hearing is processed in the *temporal lobes,* located on the sides of the brain near the temples. Most short-term memory resides in the temporal lobes, but more permanent memories do not appear to be localized to one region in the brain. *Wernicke's area,* which is involved with understanding language, is also found in the temporal cortex.

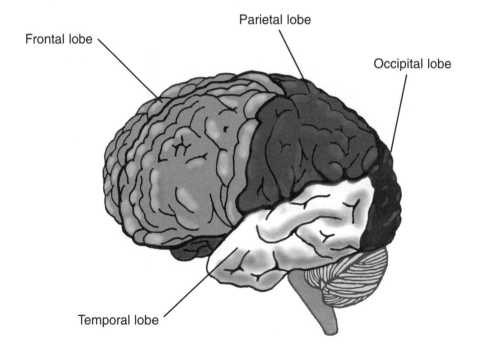

**Figure 2.2. The Cerebral Lobes**

The *parietal lobes,* tucked between the frontal and temporal lobes toward the back of the cortex, deal with spatial and sensory perception. Information processed here allows us to orient ourselves to our environment. Because of their centralized position, the parietal lobes relay information to and from the other lobes and make associations between incoming stimuli and stored memories. In addition, the parietal lobes orchestrate communication between the brain and the rest of the body.

The *occipital lobes,* small areas near the base of the brain, process vision. If this area of your brain were damaged, vision would be lost, even if your eyes were intact.

**The Limbic System**

Surrounding the top of the brain stem is an area known as the *limbic system.* "Limbus" means border, and the limbic system consists of interconnected regions in the center of the brain. The limbic system governs feelings. Maternal instincts, sexual behavior, feeding and fighting instincts, aggression, fear, pleasure, and pain all originate in the limbic system. It also, along with other areas of the brain, plays an important role in memory, which explains why so many of our most powerful memories involve strong emotions. The limbic system is composed of four primary parts— the thalamus, hypothalamus, amygdala, and hippocampus.

The *thalamus* receives all sensory impulses, with the exception of smell (which has its own center in the olfactory bulb), and relays them to specialized areas in the cortex for further processing. It also relays motor messages from the motor cortex of the cerebrum. Pain sensations are processed in the thalamus, and it is thus considered the body's "pain center."

The *hypothalamus,* although only the size of a pea, has multiple functions. It regulates the sympathetic and parasympathetic nervous systems, which control the automatic, involuntary functions of the heart, glands, and smooth muscle tissues. It is also involved in the regulation of body temperature, hunger, fluid balance, sugar and fat metabolism, sexual drive, and mating behavior. In addition, the hypothalamus is the gatekeeper of the endocrine system, as it feeds information to the pituitary gland, which, in turn,

## Does Brain Size Matter?

Remember *ET? Close Encounters of the Third Kind?* The one constant in the physical description of the intellectually superior aliens that populate science fiction is a big head. Among species on earth, there is indeed a relationship between brain size and intelligence. The bigger the brain, the smarter the species—but only when brain size is measured in relation to total body weight. An elephant, for example, has a bigger brain than a human does, but its massive body size offsets the overall proportion. Humans are the most intelligent beings on the planet, and although our brains aren't the largest pound for pound, they make up the largest percentage of total weight.

Before those of you with a large hat size puff up too much, within the human species, brain size appears to have little effect on intellect. Russian novelist Ivan Turgenev had a huge brain—4.4 pounds compared to the average 3 pounds. Yet Albert Einstein's brain was of average size, and the brain of Anatole France, who won the Nobel prize in literature, weighed in at a measly 2.2 pounds.

orchestrates other glands and hormones. The *amygdala* is linked to those areas of the brain involved in sensory perception and emotional response. It helps process emotion-laden memories and determines the emotional context of thoughts.

The *hippocampus* is a part of the brain that we'll return to often in discussions of memory and learning. It processes sensory input and acts as a sort of relay station in the brain, discarding some things, keeping a few as short-term memories, and routing others to long-term memory storage in other areas of the brain. Injury to the hippocampus interferes with the retention of new memories. The hippocampus also houses spatial memory—your brain's navigational system. It is one of the areas of the brain that is affected early in Alzheimer's disease, which explains why Alzheimer's patients have problems with short-term memory, and why they sometimes wander off and get lost.

## THE BRAIN'S IMMUNE SYSTEM

Even though they outnumber nerve cells in the brain, *glial cells* (or *neuroglia*) have long been dismissed as little more than the supporting structure of the brain and nervous system. (Glia comes from the Greek word for glue.) New research reveals that some glial cells, particularly *microglia,* act as the brain's immune system.

Because your brain is a very sensitive, specialized organ, it needs to be protected from many of the potentially harmful substances circulating in the blood. A membrane of cellular and chemical sentries, known as the *blood-brain barrier,* controls what goes into and out of the brain and cerebrospinal fluid. Although this barrier lets in selected agents of your body's immune system, for the most part, your brain must fend for itself. This underscores the importance of the brain's own immune defense system.

The glial cells involved in immunity in the brain behave much like other immune system cells, attacking invaders, surrounding injured or dying neurons, and—as an inevitable side effect of these protective actions—producing inflammatory and other damaging chemicals. It is now believed that overactive glial cells and their production of harmful chemicals may be a factor in some neurological disorders, including Alzheimer's disease.

## THE WIRING OF THE BRAIN

The "brains" of the brain are *neurons.* As seen in Figure 2.3, neurons are single cells that consist of a cell body containing the *nucleus* of the cell, an elongated fiber called the *axon,* and varying numbers of branching fibers called *dendrites.* Most axons are sheathed in *myelin,* a fat and protein coating that insulates and protects them and significantly speeds up the transmission of electrical impulses. The terminal ends of axons send messages, and the dendrites receive them. Dendrites, which can number in the tens to hundreds of thousands for each neuron, form intricate communications networks throughout the brain.

A single thought requires the activation of an entire network of neurons, whose elongated, treelike shape makes them particularly adept at communicating with other neurons. First, an electric impulse signals an axon into action. Small vesicles or sacs on the terminal end containing chemicals called *neurotransmitters* burst open and release these neurotransmitters across the *synapse* or *synaptic gap* or *cleft*, the small space between the sending and receiving cells. The neurotransmitter molecules attach to receptors on the dendrites of the adjacent neuron and cause it to "fire" and carry the electrical impulse down its axon. In a similar fashion, the impulse is then carried to the next neuron in a bioelectrical chain reaction until it reaches the target area.

Once the transaction is completed, the neurotransmitter is either reabsorbed by the neuron that initially released it, or it is inactivated by enzymes or glial cells. Strings of these neuronal transmissions working together make up what is called a *memory trace*. They interconnect different areas of the brain and allow associations between specialized areas of the brain to be made. Every time you try a new task, meet an unfamiliar person, or listen to a new song, new connections are made by these same basic neuronal axon-to-dendrite, domino-like chain reactions.

Exactly how neurons hang on to memories is uncertain. It is believed that there is a physical alteration in the RNA of the cells, perhaps in the form of encoded proteins. There is also a biochemical change at the synapses involving calcium, the neuro-

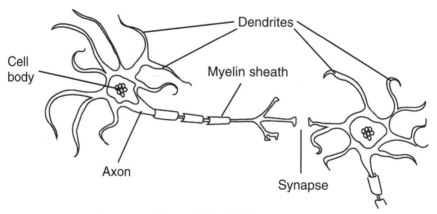

**Figure 2.3. A Neuron**

transmitter glutamate, and the amino acid N-methyl-D-aspartate (NMDA). Regardless of the exact mechanisms involved, we do know that the more times a particular neuronal pathway is stimulated, the stronger it becomes. Dendrites branch out and make stronger connections; in this way, thoughts and memories become "wired in." It appears that the concept of "use it or lose it," which we associate with muscles and physical exercise, pertains to synaptic connections and mental exercise or thinking as well. (More on this in Step 6 of the program.)

The complexity of the whole process is overwhelming and defies description. According to noted neurologist Richard Restak, M.D., author of *Brainscapes,* there are millions of billions of these neuronal connections in your brain!

## NEUROTRANSMITTERS: YOUR CHEMICAL MESSENGERS

Let's take a closer look at neurotransmitters, the chemicals that spill out of the axon of one neuron, jump across the synaptic gap between two neurons, and carry information to the dendrites of the second neuron. Because they are the chemical messengers of the brain, neurotransmitters have a profound effect on overall brain functioning. There are dozens, perhaps hundreds of neurotransmitters, many of which have yet to be studied adequately. Let's take a look at a few of those most integral to brain function.

One of the most important and abundant neurotransmitters in the brain is *acetylcholine,* which has a vital role in the processes of learning and memory. It is concentrated in the hippocampus, where memories are processed. The production of acetylcholine is severely decreased in people with Alzheimer's disease, and most of the current drug therapies for Alzheimer's attempt to raise its levels.

Another important neurotransmitter is *gamma-aminobutyric acid (GABA).* GABA is known as an inhibitory or calming neurotransmitter because it controls the firing of nerve impulses that could otherwise literally overwhelm the brain with too many stimuli. This is especially important in this age of information overload; it's what keeps us from overreacting to constant sensory bombardment. In fact, low levels of GABA are associated with chronic anxiety, and a major class of anti-anxiety drugs, the benzodiazapines (including tranquilizers such as Valium), target GABA receptor sites in the brain.

While GABA calms the brain, other neurotransmitters energize and stimulate it. One stimulating or excitatory neurotransmitter is the amino acid *glutamate*. It is present in many areas of the brain and activates systems involved with memory, thought, motor skills, and perception. Together with GABA and other inhibitory neurotransmitters, glutamate helps keep the brain on an even keel. *Dopamine* is another neurotransmitter that has a stimulating effect on the brain. It is also involved in mood, memory, and sex drive, as well as control of movement—particularly fine-motor coordination. When dopamine levels fall to a critical low, Parkinson's disease results, with its characteristic tremors and coordination difficulties.

*Serotonin* is the "happy" neurotransmitter. Low levels are associated with depression. Popular antidepressants, including Prozac and other selective serotonin reuptake inhibitors (SSRIs), are designed to boost serotonin levels by slowing down the reab-

## The Electricity of the Brain

Electricity is the engine of the brain. An electrical impulse is what prompts the release or "spilling" of neurotransmitters at the synapses and moves the thought along the axon. Brain waves, as measured by an electroencephalogram (EEG), are nothing more than electrical impulses within the brain.

Certain types of brain waves are associated with specific mental activities. For example, the slowest, most dominant wave pattern during sleep is *delta*. In the normal waking state, *beta*, the highest frequency waves, predominate. *Alpha* waves are common in relaxed states. During periods of meditation or intense concentration, problem solving, and creativity, *theta* waves prevail. We'll talk more about brain waves in the discussion on sleep in Step 8 of the program.

sorption of serotonin by the cells. Serotonin is also involved in sleep, appetite control, and pain control.

*Norepinephrine,* also called *noradrenaline,* is a stimulating neurotransmitter that keeps you alert. It is also produced in the adrenal glands in response to stress. Norepinephrine is also crucial in memory as it helps embed long-term memories. That's why we remember exciting, scary, painful events better than run-of-the-mill happenings. It's important for survival to remember that putting your hand in the fire or rushing into traffic is not a good thing. But too much norepinephrine impedes the storage of memories and interferes with proper brain function, which is one reason why chronic stress is very harmful to the brain.

*Endorphins* are neurotransmitters produced in response to stress. They blunt some of the negative effects of stress—dulling pain perception, reducing anxiety, and producing a sensation of pleasure. Maybe you are familiar with the sense of euphoria that results from exercise, such as the "runner's high." Because exercise is a form of physical stress, it releases a flood of feel-good endorphins.

## THE BRAIN IS PART OF AN INTEGRATED SYSTEM

While I have given you a rather mechanical overview of the brain and its components, I do not want to give the impression that the brain is a separate entity, presiding over the rest of the body from above. Nothing could be further from the truth. Your body is an integrated whole. Your endocrine, cardiovascular, and other organ systems, as well as lifestyle factors such as diet, exercise, and stress levels, all have a tremendous influence on brain function.

Great strides have been made in recent years in understanding the workings of the brain and its interrelationships with other organs and functions of the body. Chronic stress doesn't just make you feel tired and edgy, it damages brain cells. We now know that a diet loaded with sugar and unhealthy fats not only puts on the pounds and increases your risk of heart disease, it also starves your brain of needed nutrients. In addition to improving muscle strength and cardiovascular endurance, exercise enhances every aspect of your health, including your cognitive function.

In the next chapter, you will see how these various factors affect your brain. We'll look at how the brain ages and explore the medical conditions, drugs, and environmental and lifestyle factors that accelerate this process, resulting in memory loss and cognitive dysfunction. Then we'll move on to Part Two and explore the specific steps you can take to sharpen your memory and mental edge.

# CHAPTER 3

# Your Brain at Risk

*M*ary had an illustrious career as a high-level secretary with the Department of Defense, spoke several languages, and lived in Europe for several years while on assignment. When she was sixty-five, she left her job and moved to a retirement community in Arizona where she played golf three times a week and was actively involved in church activities.

*Although Mary had had high blood pressure for many years, she had no real health challenges until her early seventies, when she suffered a series of small strokes. Although she appeared to recover, her family was concerned. When they called Mary, she seemed "spacy." This bright, articulate woman repeated herself, searched for words, and was often unable to recall a conversation held just the day before. This went on for months until the family got a call from the emergency room of the local hospital saying that Mary was in the emergency room for burns from a minor kitchen fire that had started when she accidentally left a burner on.*

*It was clear that Mary could no longer live on her own, and her niece, Darlene, offered her a room in her house. For the next five years, Mary lived with her niece's family in California. In the beginning, she was an engaging companion, generally lucid, with memory lapses that were more humorous than anything else. But by the third year, Mary's lapses outweighed her lucid moments, and she could no longer be left alone. Still, even though it was becoming a burden and strain on her family, Darlene was reluctant to relinquish the care of her beloved aunt.*

*After five years, however, Darlene realized that she could no longer handle Mary. Even when she was attended, Mary would manage to get out of the house and wander off, causing hours of worry until she was found. She was also beginning to be verbally abusive to Darlene and her two sons. She practically had to be forced to eat, and, most difficult, she was becoming incontinent.*

*Darlene eventually placed Mary in a nursing home, where she lingered for two years, becoming increasingly less aware and more passive until she died. Not surprisingly, an autopsy revealed that Mary had Alzheimer's disease.*

Although Alzheimer's is considered an illness of the brain, as Mary's story poignantly illustrates, it ravages the body, mind, and soul. In this age of medical specialization, when cardiologists handle hearts and hearts only, orthopedists treat bones exclusively, and the brain is the guarded domain of neurologists and psychiatrists, the patient as an integrated whole is often overlooked. The conventional view of medicine tends to view the patient as a grouping of body parts with unrelated symptoms and diagnoses. As a result, physicians prescribe drugs for diabetes that lower blood sugar but may increase the risk of heart disease. They give patients with arthritis painkillers that cause gastrointestinal bleeding. They subject patients to surgical procedures that temporarily open an artery or reduce the size of the prostate—but may have long-lasting detrimental effects on other aspects of the patient's well-being.

This is the antithesis of the type of medicine I practice. Good medicine, in my opinion, requires a holistic view of the human body, and putting the brain or any organ system in its own separate little box disregards this important concept. What affects one part of the body affects the whole.

What I want to make clear in this chapter is that there are deeper explanations of disease processes that cause declines in physical, mental, and emotional health. Some of them, of course, are beyond your control. You cannot change your genes, subtract years from your age, or reverse a past history of poor lifestyle choices, such as smoking or drinking heavily. However, you may be surprised by the degree to which the things you choose to do every day—what you eat, what drugs and nutritional supplements you take, how you manage your stress and activity levels—impact your cognitive function and overall health.

While I will target only those risk factors that are known to specifically affect the brain, it is important that you realize that the majority of these factors are involved in other disease processes, particularly the degenerative diseases associated with aging. Thus, by following the 10-step program presented in Part Two, you'll improve not only your memory and brainpower, but your overall health as well. Your blood pressure and cholesterol will likely drop, thus reducing your risk of stroke and heart disease. Your chances of developing diabetes will decrease, and your weight may normalize. Your bone mass will improve, and your risk of osteoporosis will fall. Because these general therapeutic principles address both your mental faculties and physical health, you will likely find yourself with increased strength, endurance, and flexibility.

## AGING—THE GREATEST RISK FACTOR

The single greatest contributor to memory loss and cognitive decline is aging. The aging of the brain is part and parcel of the overall aging process. However, it doesn't happen overnight. You don't just wake up at the age of sixty-five or seventy with an old brain and a lousy memory. If you pay attention, you'll notice gradual changes—perhaps increasing forgetfulness or problems with word and name recall. Unfortunately, most people ignore these small changes and minor deficits. They just live with them. What a difference it would make if we would tune into our bodies, heed the subtle warning signs of impending disease and degeneration, and take proactive steps towards better health early in life. I have no doubt that we could stave off the aging process, increase life span, and, more important, dramatically improve health and quality of life throughout all of our years.

What is aging exactly, other than the passage of years? We used to just take it for granted that aging involves the systemic breakdown of the body, but we never really understood how this happened. Now a solid and growing body of scientific research has identified a general framework—four major categories of interrelated biological changes that contribute to the degenerative diseases associated with aging and the aging process itself. These four processes, which have been neatly tied together by Dr. Jeffrey Bland, director of the Institute for Functional Medicine in Gig Harbor, Washington, offer the most comprehensive rationale for why our brains and bodies deteriorate as we age. They are oxidative or free-radical damage, glycation, inflammation, and methylation defects.

## Oxidative Damage

*Oxidative* or *free-radical damage* is the dominant theory of why we age. Free radicals, which are byproducts of normal cellular metabolism, are highly reactive atoms or molecules that bind to and destroy healthy cells. Breathing, extracting energy from food—just living—creates free radicals. Your cells' energy-producing factories, the *mitochondria,* and mitochondrial DNA are at special risk for free-radical damage. And once energy production slows down, everything slows down. Fat cells are also at high risk for oxidation, and because the brain has such a high concentration of fat (60 percent), it is exceptionally vulnerable to oxidation.

Your body has an elaborate system of *antioxidants* to neutralize free radicals and fight the damage caused by oxidation. However, years of accumulated free-radical damage, accelerated by the realities of modern life that increase oxidative stress (environmental pollution, smoking, eating fried foods, stress, etc.), take a tremendous toll on the body. This leads to all kinds of degenerative diseases, including heart disease, circulatory problems, arthritis, and Alzheimer's disease, as well as loss of cellular energy and organ reserve. The eventual result is a complete system breakdown. Dietary and supplemental antioxidants, which are discussed in Steps 1 and 2 of the program, help counteract free radicals and protect against these degenerative changes.

## Glycation

The aptly named *advanced glycation end products (AGEs)* are another aging factor. AGEs are formed when proteins in the body react with excess glucose, or blood sugar, your body's primary energy source. This process is known as *glycation* and results in these chemically damaged and altered proteins. AGEs accumulate in the tissues, causing damage to the immune, nervous, and endocrine systems. They are particularly problematic in people with blood sugar abnormalities, such as diabetes and insulin resistance—a "pre-diabetic" condition that is estimated to affect 25 percent of the population and is increasingly common with advancing age. AGEs are also implicated in diabetic complications of the eyes, circulatory system, and kidneys. Glycation is a known factor in Alzheimer's disease.

Keeping insulin and blood sugar levels in check may slow the progress of glycation and the development of age-related degeneration. As discussed in Step 1 of the program, diet is an important factor in the control of glycation.

## Inflammation

Part of your immune system's reaction to injury or attack from bacteria or other harmful agents is *inflammation*. This complex reaction is set in motion to protect the site of injury or infection and promote healing. Small blood vessels in the injured area dilate, and swelling or edema may develop as blood vessels leak fluid. Immune cells rush to the area, and fibrin and other blood-clotting agents are formed. This is an essential part of the healing process and is short-lived in most cases. As we get older, however, and our circulation becomes sluggish from years of plaque buildup on artery walls, our ability to remove the byproducts of inflammation is impaired. Furthermore, the signaling mechanisms of the immune system get sloppy, and our own healthy tissue is sometimes misidentified as foreign and is attacked. The result is chronic inflammation.

Recent research has found links between chronic inflammation and a variety of age-related diseases, including cardiovascular disease, autoimmune disorders, arthritis, dementia, and Alzheimer's disease. The Alzheimer's connection is particularly strong, and autopsies of brains afflicted with this disease show signs of inflammation. Therefore, it is likely that measures to control chronic inflammation, including the selection of healthy fats in the diet and specific nutritional supplements discussed in Part Two, may slow down the aging process and improve brain function.

## Methylation Defects

Methylation is your body's chief mechanism for internal detoxification. It is, in a sense, cellular housecleaning, and without it harmful compounds build up. One of these compounds is *homocysteine,* a byproduct of normal amino acid metabolism.

Homocysteine becomes toxic when it is present in the body in high levels. It impairs circulation, as it encourages the platelets in the blood to stick together. This results in thick, sludge-like blood. It also stimulates free-radical damage, damages the cells' DNA, and initiates and accelerates atherosclerosis, heart disease, cancer, Alzheimer's disease, and other degenerative conditions. Homocysteine levels are abnormally high in most patients with Alzheimer's disease.

## Hormones and Aging

Another important factor in aging is the decline in your body's production of hormones. You all know how drops in estrogen trigger menopause in women, but you may not know that men undergo similar, although less abrupt, reductions in testosterone production. Beginning in your forties or fifties (precisely the time during which the aging process speeds up), levels of these and other hormones—thyroid, melatonin, progesterone, DHEA, and pregnenolone—begin to decline. These hormonal changes have tremendous effects on your physical health and cognitive function. Supplementing with certain hormones, as discussed in Step 9 of the program, will help protect your body and brain from the ravages of aging.

Defects in methylation are common as we age, as are elevated levels of homocysteine. In order for the methylation process to run smoothly and homocysteine to be kept at manageable levels, adequate amounts of folic acid and vitamin $B_{12}$ must be present. Vitamin $B_6$ is also involved in a peripheral role. Making sure you get adequate amounts of these nutrients will keep your body's methylation process in tiptop condition.

## STRESS IS A MIND-KILLER

Chronic stress contributes to memory loss and mental dysfunction. Regardless of whether the source is physical or emotional, real or imagined, there is a definite physiological, biochemical response to stress. It is a carryover from the "fight-or-flight" response to stress that was necessary for survival in our ancestors' world of physical dangers. Your system is bathed in hormones and chemicals that prepare you mentally and physically to do battle or run like hell.

Animal studies have demonstrated that prolonged stress and exposure to high levels of stress hormones called *glucocorticoids* (which include *cortisol*) damage the brain and accelerate brain aging. Cortisol is particularly hard on the hippocampus, the area of the brain involved in learning and memory. And it appears to have similar effects in humans. A five-year study done at McGill University in Montreal, Canada, periodically measured the blood levels of stress hormones in 130 healthy people between the ages of fifty-five and eighty-seven. In these individuals, high levels of stress hormones were associated with memory and attention deficits. Elevated levels of cortisol have even been proposed as a cause of Alzheimer's disease.

In addition, depression often accompanies uncontrolled stress, and depression is responsible for perhaps 10 percent of all cases of memory impairment. Stress typically contributes to sleep disturbances, which also affect memory and cognitive function. One of the best things you can do to protect your brain and enhance your cognitive functioning is get a handle on stress. Step 7 offers helpful tips on how to do this.

## ENVIRONMENTAL TOXINS THAT AFFECT THE BRAIN

Another contributor to brain aging and dysfunction is exposure to *neurotoxins,* environmental elements, such as heavy metals and pesticides, and certain food additives and pharmaceutical drugs that negatively affect the brain and the nervous system. Many neurotoxins are *xenobiotics* (*xenos* means "stranger" in Greek), manmade chemicals that negatively affect the biological systems of animals and humans. Every day we are exposed to hundreds of these chemicals.

Neurotoxicity is a diagnostic quagmire. Since it doesn't show up on conventional testing, symptoms such as confusion, memory loss, and fatigue can easily be attributed to other causes, and most physicians are simply unaware of the profound effects environmental elements may have on health. However, neurotoxicity is a growing concern. A few years ago, while examining environmental pollutants, a U.S. Government Subcommittee on Investigations and Oversight concluded that neurotoxins were one of the country's top ten causes of illness.

There is an ever-growing list of environmental toxins that may temporarily or permanently affect the brain. These include pesticides, herbicides, and solvents or other cleaning agents. Among the most dangerous are certain heavy metals, food additives, and drugs.

### Heavy Metals

One of the most prevalent neurotoxins is *lead.* Acute lead exposure is a well-documented cause of brain and nervous system damage and mental retardation, especially in children. It is likely that even low levels of this toxic metal also have harmful effects. Environmental sources of lead include tap water (many older plumbing systems use lead-soldered pipes), lead-soldered cans (once they're opened, lead immediately begins to leach into the can's contents), lead-based paint (although banned in the 1980s, this type of paint is still out there), crystal (fine crystal may contain up to 30-percent lead oxide), and some ceramic and earthenware containers (many are decorated with colorful lead-based glazes). And even though lead in gasoline has been banned since 1972, our soils contain deadly accumulations of this neurotoxin from years of automobile emissions.

Another common neurotoxin is *aluminum.* Autopsies of the brains of patients with Alzheimer's disease consistently reveal high levels of aluminum in brain tissue. At this time, however, this finding is like the chicken-or-egg hypothesis—which came first? We don't know whether these metal concentrations actually *cause* the disease or are somehow deposited in the brain as a *result* of the disease. However, support for the causative role of aluminum in Alzheimer's disease is growing. Studies have found relationships between aluminum levels in drinking water and Alzheimer's disease, with up to a 250-percent increased risk with the highest aluminum levels. Aluminum cookware, antiperspirants, beverage cans, and baking powder are the primary sources of ingested aluminum. Inhaled aluminum, particularly from spray-on antiperspirants, is particularly worrisome, as the olfactory receptors in the nose shuttle inhaled molecules directly into the brain.

*Mercury* is yet another neurotoxic heavy metal. A number of incidents have been recorded in which mercury that had been inadvertently released into the environment caused widespread poisoning and severe brain damage. Because it is such a well-recognized neurotoxin, mercury is kept under tight wraps, except for one common usage: dental fillings. Despite the stubborn insistence on its safety by the American Dental Association, there is a growing body of research that clearly shows mercury in dental amalgam fillings to be anything but innocuous. I personally have had all my amalgam fillings removed and replaced with safer materials.

## Food Additives and Allergens

Certain food additives cause cognitive impairment in some people, and, in high enough doses, these chemicals are believed to be toxic to virtually everyone. Two particularly problematic food additives are monosodium glutamate (MSG) and aspartame (NutraSweet). They will be discussed in detail in Step 1 of the program.

To avoid ingesting harmful additives, eat food as close to its natural state as possible, and buy organic produce when available. Be aware that for people with food allergies, even common foods can be neurotoxic. Food allergies are a big issue—and one that is seldom addressed—in cases of hyperactivity and attention deficit disorder. I've seen bright, well-behaved children become inattentive and out of control simply from eating foods to which they are allergic. Similar reactions to allergens may occur in adults.

## Drugs

Many drugs are poisonous to the brain. It goes without saying that recreational drugs like cocaine and amphetamines are extremely dangerous and can have far-reaching effects on the brain's chemistry. Antidepressants, tranquilizers, and barbiturates are designed to alter brain function, and they do so at the expense of memory and alertness. Many other commonly taken drugs, including beta-blockers, calcium channel blockers, painkillers, and antihistamines, also interfere with brain function. The following list includes a number of drugs that can cause memory problems.

| | |
|---|---|
| Antidepressants | Glaucoma eye drops |
| Antihistamines | Incontinence medications |
| Antipsychotics | Muscle relaxants |
| Barbiturates | Painkillers |
| Beta-blockers | Sedatives |
| Calcium channel blockers | Sleeping pills |
| Digitalis | Tranquilizers |

The more drugs you take, the greater the likelihood of memory problems. Even when drugs are used as prescribed, adverse reactions are extremely common. According to a 1998 report published in the *Journal of the American Medical Association*, prescription drugs take the lives of an estimated 106,000 Americans each year. In addition, as we get older, our sensitivity to drugs may change. What is a safe dose for a younger person may be toxic to someone older. Take a careful look at your medication list, and work with your doctor to see which drugs, if any, you might be able to cut back on or gradually eliminate.

## Smoking

Nicotine improves concentration and memory. Ask any smoker. There are actually nicotinic receptors in your brain to which both nicotine and acetylcholine, the neurotransmitter involved in memory and learning, bind. Nicotine facilitates communication among the neurons and increases the production of neurotransmitters. There have even been reports that smokers are at reduced risk for Alzheimer's disease, and nicotine patches have been successfully used on patients with this disease to improve memory.

On the other hand, smoking damages your body in more ways than you could possibly imagine. It's well known that smoking puts you at an increased risk for lung cancer and cardiovascular disease. It also alters brainwave patterns and causes an increase in stress hormone levels, including brain-damaging cortisol. Processed tobacco exposes the smoker—and those around him or her—to yet another toxic heavy metal, cadmium. Smoking also severely restricts blood flow and depletes stores of available oxygen in the blood. In fact, it takes up to eight hours for blood oxygen levels to return to normal after smoking just one cigarette. This doesn't bode well for the brain, which has voracious oxygen requirements. And in fact, a 1998 study of 9,223 men and women over the age of sixty-five demonstrated that smokers have more rapid mental decline, compared to nonsmokers.

Scientists are exploring the use of nicotine—not smoking—as a brain booster. If you're a smoker, quit. It's the single most important lifestyle change you can implement to improve your health.

## Alcohol

An occasional alcoholic drink won't hurt most people, and, in fact, numerous studies have demonstrated that judicious use of alcohol (one or two drinks per day or less) provides protection against heart disease. There has even been a study conducted in France suggesting that moderate alcohol intake actually enhances cognitive performance in older women. (Alcohol gave men no edge in similar tests that measured learning, language, and problem-solving skills.)

Heavy alcohol use is another thing altogether. Alcohol destroys brain cells, and chronic heavy drinking causes permanent damage to the brain. Long-term alcoholism is associated with a condition called *Korsakoff's psychosis*, which is characterized by severe short- and long-term memory loss. Even infrequent, episodic heavy drinking can damage the brain and diminish memory and cognitive performance for hours following the binge. Animal studies reveal that the damage from heavy alcohol use is most extensive to the hippocampus, the brain's memory processing center. If you choose to drink alcohol, be sure to do so in moderation.

## STROKE AND OTHER INJURY TO THE BRAIN

Injury to the brain can produce deficits in thinking, behavior, and/or mood. Brain injury refers not only to physical trauma to the head, but also to secondary injury resulting from disease processes such as stroke. Because the brain is so specialized, injury to different areas results in varying, sometimes bizarre, deficits. If the language center in the temporal lobe is injured, speech is affected. Damage to the cerebellum, which controls movement, may cause muscular disorders. Problems in the occipital lobe may affect vision.

Neurologist Oliver Sacks, in his fascinating book, *The Man Who Mistook His Wife for a Hat*, relates several stories of patients with unusual mental deficits caused by damage to the brain. The case history from which the book draws its title concerns Dr. P., a musician and music teacher who suffered internal brain damage. Although Dr. P. maintained normal overall functioning, including his musical ability and sense of humor, he was unable to "see" faces. Once someone spoke to him, he recognized the person, but he simply could not perceive his or her face.

# Reversible Memory Robbers

Memory loss, including severe memory loss, frequently can be reversed by addressing underlying, yet often overlooked, causes. Some of these causes include:

• **Depression.** Approximately 10 percent of all people with memory loss and mental impairment are depressed. Once this condition is treated and mood is elevated, memory may be restored. Step 7 of the program discusses natural remedies for depression.

• **Vitamin B$_{12}$ deficiency.** This common deficiency is the cause of as much as one-third of the mental deterioration and confusion in older people. It can be remedied by B$_{12}$ supplementation, as discussed in Step 2 of the program.

• **Adverse drug reactions.** A number of drugs have been identified as contributors to memory loss (see page 46 for a partial listing). Speak to your doctor about possible adverse drug reactions, especially if you are taking multiple prescriptions.

Other treatable medical conditions, such as structural lesions in the brain (benign tumors, subdural hematomas), infections of the brain or nervous system, and metabolic imbalances (high or low thyroid or sodium concentrations), may also be sources of cognitive dysfunction. These conditions should be ruled out by a qualified medical professional.

Furthermore, he "saw faces where there were no faces to see," on parking meters, water hydrants, and the like.

One of the most common types of injury to the brain is a *stroke* (also called *brain infarct, cerebrovascular accident,* or *brain attack*), which harms the brain by disrupting its oxygen supply. A stroke occurs when an artery in the brain bursts or becomes completely clogged, cutting off oxygen to an area of the brain. Brain cells in the oxygen-deprived area begin dying within minutes. Patients who have suffered a stroke have varying degrees of brain damage. Impairments in speech and coordination are perhaps the most common symptoms in the aftermath of a stroke, and in many cases they are temporary. But severe strokes can result in permanent paralysis, a multitude of deficits, even death. It has recently been discovered that repeated multiple small strokes—even those so minor they are not noticeable at the time of occurrence—are a significant risk factor for Alzheimer's disease. A 1997 study, based on the autopsies of 102 nuns, found that small strokes were an important contributor to the development of Alzheimer's disease.

Stroke is a chief cause of disability and the third leading cause of death in the United States. Common warning signs include sudden vision impairment, dizziness, weakness on one side of the body, confusion, numbness and paralysis, loss of bowel or bladder control, severe headache, and loss of consciousness. Identifying and treating a stroke at once is vitally important, as most brain damage occurs in the first few hours following the stroke. The best way to approach stroke is to take measures to avoid having one. High blood pressure is a high risk factor for strokes, as are atrial fibrillation (irregular heartbeat), diabetes, smoking, and use of oral contraceptives. The diet; vitamin, mineral, and herbal supplementation; and exercise recommendations in Part Two provide protection against strokes by normalizing blood pressure and improving cardiovascular health.

## MEDICAL CONDITIONS THAT PROMOTE NEURODEGENERATION

Alzheimer's disease is the medical condition most frequently associated with damage to or degeneration of the brain, with resulting cognitive dysfunction. However, there are several other common medical conditions not generally associated with the brain that are known to increase the risk of memory loss and dementia.

### Atherosclerosis

Atherosclerosis is the thickening, hardening, and loss of elasticity of the blood vessels, particularly the arteries. It is accompanied by a buildup of plaque that reduces the diameter of the blood vessels and decreases blood flow throughout the body, including the brain. Your brain requires a continuous supply of glucose and oxygen, which are delivered to your brain by the blood. When blood flow is limited, as it may be with atherosclerosis of the carotid arteries (the two large arteries on either side of your neck that supply blood to the brain), your brain suffers. People with this condition, which is known as carotid artery stenosis, are at greater risk for stroke. Their odds are also greater for *transient ischemic attacks (TIAs)*, also referred to as mini-strokes, and general memory deficits.

Atherosclerosis is common as we age, but it can be minimized and even reversed by implementing a low-fat diet, exercise, and, perhaps most important, an aggressive regimen of high-dose nutritional supplements, as discussed in Step 2 of the program.

## High Blood Pressure

High blood pressure, or hypertension, endangers your brain in several ways. First, it is associated with atherosclerosis and significantly increased risk of stroke, both of which are factors in mental deterioration. But hypertension also appears to be a risk factor for cognitive dysfunction in itself. A study published in 1995, funded by the National Institute on Aging, examined the relationships between hypertension and cognitive function. Over 4,000 Japanese-American men living in Hawaii were followed for twenty-five years. During that time, periodic physical examinations were performed and medical histories were kept. When these men were given a test of cognitive function at the average age of seventy-eight, it was discovered that the risk of poor cognitive function at this age was progressively associated with the degree of hypertension the men had experienced in mid-life. In other words, the men most likely to score poorly on mental function testing were those who had high blood pressure twenty-five years earlier.

Researchers at the National Institute on Aging confirmed these findings. They compared people who had well-controlled high blood pressure in two age groups—fifty-six to sixty-nine and seventy to eighty-four—with those who had normal blood pressure. These hypertensive patients were able to keep their blood pressures within the normal range with the help of medication and other measures, and none had had a stroke or other medical problems. However, compared to the people with normal blood pressure, the patients with hypertension—in both the younger and older groups—had significantly increased atrophy, or shrinkage, of the brain, as well as more severe memory loss, which worsened with age.

Like atherosclerosis, hypertension may be improved and your risk of stroke and brain atrophy lowered by dietary and lifestyle measures, including those discussed in Steps 1 and 2 of the program.

## Diabetes Mellitus

Diabetes is a disorder of carbohydrate metabolism. Those with type I diabetes, also known as juvenile or insulin-dependent diabetes, experience elevated blood sugar levels because their bodies do not produce adequate insulin—the storage hormone that ushers blood sugar into the cells. In the absence of sufficient amounts of insulin, blood sugar cannot enter the cells and it climbs to dangerously high levels. Fortunately, this type of diabetes affects only a small portion of all diabetics. Over 90 percent of diabetics have type II diabetes, also known as adult-onset or non-insulin-dependent diabetes mellitus (NIDDM). Most people with NIDDM produce enough insulin, but their bodies are unable to utilize it correctly, a condition known as *insulin resistance.*

Diabetes is hard on the body. Elevated blood sugar and insulin levels damage blood vessels, impair circulation, and injure the eyes, kidneys, and nerves. Furthermore, NIDDM is associated with a 30-percent increase in dementia, according to a Dutch study presented at the 1996 annual meeting of the American Academy of Neurology. Researchers looked at 6,330 residents of a Rotterdam suburb who were at least fifty-five years old. Of the 11.4 percent who had diabetes, 22.3 percent experienced dementia or mental deterioration, compared to only 11 percent of the non-diabetic population. Dr. Monique M. Breteler, one of the study's principal investigators, stated, "Apart from the obvious lesions caused by strokes, subtle neurochemical, electrophysiologic, and structural changes have been found in the brains of patients with NIDDM."

Although type I diabetes must be treated with insulin, the more common adult-onset type (NIDDM) responds well to exercise, dietary changes, and targeted nutritional supplements.

## Brain Tumors

Brain tumors, whether benign or malignant, invade the brain and impinge on brain tissue, impeding its function. Malignant brain tumors are, as a rule, especially fast growing and virulent, and the patient's prognosis is usually grave. As in all cancers, chemotherapy and radiation are the primary treatments, but they are largely ineffective in brain cancer, and the damage the therapies themselves cause makes the treatment sometimes more of a nightmare than the disease.

It is not my intent to offer a discourse on brain cancer, but because the traditional therapies are so ineffective and the prognosis for patients with brain malignancies so dismal, I want to make you aware of one "alternative" therapy. Stanislaw Burzynski, M.D., of Houston, Texas, has discovered what I consider to be the biggest breakthrough in cancer treatment of this century—*antineoplastons*. Antineoplastons are small, naturally occurring, nontoxic particles that enter cells and alter their genetic programming. They either turn off oncogenes, which cause cancer cells to proliferate, or activate tumor suppressor genes, which stop cancer from growing. Dr. Burzynski has discovered a way to synthesize antineoplastons in the lab. He has had a growing number of documented clinical successes with this therapy, and his most consistent results have been with brain malignancies. The Burzynski Clinic is located in Houston, Texas. See the Resource Section beginning on page 255 for more information.

## ALZHEIMER'S DISEASE

The disease Americans fear most is probably Alzheimer's dis-

## Multiple Risk Factors—
## Increased Risk of Cognitive Declines

The effects of memory risk factors appear to be cumulative. The more medical conditions and negative lifestyle factors discussed in this chapter that affect you, the more likely you are to develop memory loss and cognitive impairment—and the more severe these declines are apt to be. A 1998 study, part of the ongoing Framingham Heart Study, examined the effects of high blood pressure, diabetes, obesity, and cigarette smoking on memory and thinking. Researchers found that each one of these risk factors independently lowered performance on tests of cognitive function by 23 percent—and the risk increased by 32 percent in the presence of each additional factor.

ease. I'll be the first to admit that Alzheimer's disease is scary, but except in the "oldest of the old," those eighty-five and over, it's much less common than you might think. While it's true that over 4 million Americans are afflicted with the disease, it is rare in people under fifty and uncommon in people under sixty-five. However, after the age of sixty-five, the likelihood of developing Alzheimer's doubles every five years, to almost 50 percent at age eighty-five. And as the baby boomer generation enters these older age brackets in the next few decades, the incidence of this disease is expected to quadruple.

This well-known type of dementia, first described in 1907 by German neurologist Alois Alzheimer, is a progressive disease. It develops over ten to twenty years, although generally it is not recognized in its very early stages. Alzheimer's disease is marked by a loss of neurons and significant atrophy of the brain. Characteristically, there is a critical decrease in the neurotransmitter acetylcholine, caused by degradation of the hippocampus and reduced activity of an enzyme required in the production of acetylcholine. However, the definitive markers of Alzheimer's disease, which can be determined only by a brain autopsy, are neurofibrillary tangles and neuritic plaques.

*Neurofibrillary tangles* are paired knotty filaments located inside neurons that eventually destroy the cells. *Neuritic plaques,* sometimes called senile plaques, consist of a protein core called *beta amyloid* that is surrounded by dead and dying cellular debris. The areas of the brain most rapidly affected are the hippocampus and the amygdala, areas that are important in memory processing and emotion.

Alzheimer's disease begins with short-term memory loss. But as the disease progresses and the cortex erodes, patients eventually become impulsive, agitated, and irrational, requiring full-time care. The end stages of Alzheimer's involve degeneration of the cerebellum, so basic motor skills, continence, and even the ability to self-feed are lost. This stage can last as long as seven years, and the emotional and financial tolls it takes on families are indescribable. A listing of common features of Alzheimer's disease during different stages of the illness is presented in Table 3.1.

The strongest, most definitive risk factor for Alzheimer's disease is age. As I said earlier, incidence of the disease increases after age sixty-five, and almost half of those eighty-five and older have it. Each and every one of the processes of aging—oxidation, glycation, inflammation, and methylation defects—is involved in Alzheimer's disease. Those at increased risk include females, as well as those who have experienced previous head trauma, repeated small strokes, and myocardial infarction (heart attack).

## The Genetic Link

There is a well-defined genetic link in Alzheimer's disease. It has long been apparent that a family history of Alzheimer's significantly increases your likelihood of developing the disease, but only in the last few years have we understood why. To date, four genes have been discovered that are associated with the development of Alzheimer's. Three are related to early-onset Alzheimer's, which accounts for only about 5 percent of all cases. The fourth and most common gene involves a specific allele, or pair of genes, on chromosome 19 that affects apolipoprotein E (apoE). This protein is a major component of lipoproteins—proteins that carry fats like cholesterol in the bloodstream.

### TABLE 3.1. CHARACTERISTICS OF THOSE WITH ALZHEIMER'S DISEASE

| Early Stage | Intermediate Stage | Late Stage |
|---|---|---|
| • Has poor recall of recent memories | • Has poor recall of old memories | • Has very little or no language skills |
| • Has mild loss of linguistic skills | • Has difficulty forming thoughts verbally | • Is incontinent |
| • Misplaces objects | • Has comprehension difficulties | • Is agitated |
| • Experiences mild visual/spatial deficits (may have difficulty driving, etc.) | • Is repetitious | • Wanders aimlessly |
| | • Gets lost | |
| • May have mild delusions, depression, and/or insomnia | • Has difficulty copying figures | |
| | • Experiences delusions, depression, agitation, and/or insomnia | |

People who have inherited a variation of this gene called APOE4 from each parent have a 90-percent chance of developing Alzheimer's disease by age seventy-five. According to researchers at Washington University School of Medicine in St. Louis, Missouri, and the University of Madrid in Spain, amyloid (the nucleus of senile plaque that junks up the brains of Alzheimer's patients) is deposited earlier and more easily in carriers of this genotype. Although the double APOE4 gene is a significant risk factor, it accounts for only 5 percent of the disease. The other, more controllable risk factors for Alzheimer's disease are much more important for the majority of people. Tremendous advances are being made in genetics. Someday, perhaps in the not-so-distant future, not only will we have a complete map of our genes and be able to identify the ones that put us at risk for various diseases, but we may be able to manipulate those genes and actually eliminate risk factors like this one.

I recommend that patients with Alzheimer's disease immediately begin a comprehensive program of brain nurturing, incorporating as many of the 10 steps in Part Two as possible. If you are caring for a loved one with this disease, these measures may provide added months of function. They could also have a tremendous impact on our nation's nursing homes and medical bills. If these steps delay the course of the disease and put off institutionalization by only one month, it would save the country $1.12 billion, as annual costs of institutionalizing each patient with Alzheimer's disease are upwards of $36,000 per year.

## SUMMING IT UP

This chapter has presented the risk factors that contribute to memory loss and "brain drain." Most of these factors are within your control to minimize or eliminate. Survey your home and work environment and make a list of environmental toxins that need to be eliminated. Next, look at your personal habits and see if there are any changes you need to make. By doing so, you should be able to avoid or minimize most of these potential risk factors. If you have atherosclerosis, high blood pressure, diabetes, or any other medical condition that may contribute to mental decline, use all the tools at your disposal to bring them under control—diet, exercise, nutritional supplementation, and conventional medical therapies, if necessary.

Now let's move on to Part Two—the most exciting part of this book. Here, I will lay out the 10-step program my patients have used with great success to improve their memory and retain and hone their mental edge.

# PART TWO

# 10 Steps for Sharper Memory and Mental Edge

# CHAPTER 4

## Your 10-Step Program

As you have seen in Part One, science has made great strides in understanding the human brain, including how thought and memory work and why these processes sometimes falter. Memory loss is not inevitable. And problems with memory, concentration, and other cognitive functions do not strike randomly. A number of risk factors contribute to their development, many of which are within your control. Your daily habits, the things you do on a regular basis, have significant impact on the optimal functioning of your brain.

This is great news because it puts you in the driver's seat. All it takes on your part is desire, determination, and a willingness to make a few positive adjustments in your life. The following 10-step program really works. It has been scientifically proven and successfully used by thousands of patients to improve memory and cognitive function. Equally important, this program is "doable." After decades of working with patients, I have a pretty good understanding of what people are willing to do, versus what they are not.

Although my program will require some effort on your part, I am confident that you will be able to embrace it—I guarantee it will make noticeable enhancements in your memory, concentration, problem-solving abilities, and intellect. Let's get started!

STEP 1

# Feed Your Head

*V*ivian *was a forty-eight-year-old professional, very knowledgeable about health topics, and proactive about her own health. She exercised regularly, took vitamins, and ate a low-fat diet. Yet she had difficulty concentrating and was plagued with fatigue, irritability, and mood swings. She was unable to focus at work and began letting important details slip by. After consulting her family physician, who ruled out serious medical problems, she sought my help at Whitaker Wellness Institute.*

*One of the first things I looked at, which other physicians often overlook, was Vivian's diet. She was very conscientious about what she put in her mouth; "fat" was a dirty word to her. Upon closer examination, I discovered that she was eating way too many refined carbohydrates—bagel for breakfast, sandwich for lunch, rice cakes for snacks, and potatoes or rice, and chicken or fish for dinner. I looked at the pattern of Vivian's symptoms. She felt most tired, cranky, and unfocused in the early afternoon, about an hour after lunch. I suggested that she replace bread, crackers, white rice, and potatoes with vegetables, fruit, whole grains, legumes, fish, and poultry. When she returned to the clinic a month later, Vivian reported that all of her cognitive and mood problems had vanished.*

Good nutrition is essential for optimal health and brain function, and the foundation of good nutrition is a healthy, well-balanced diet. But just what is a healthy, well-balanced diet? There is so much controversy and conflicting information on the subject of diet these days that many people simply don't know what they should eat. Some experts claim that a low-carbohydrate, high-fat diet is the way to go, while others insist on little fat and lots of carbohydrates. Many extol the virtues of a diet high in protein,

## Will Eating Less Make You Smarter?

It has long been known that eating less extends life span in animals. In fact, it's the only thing that has been proven to retard aging in mammals. In repeated experiments, laboratory animals who eat half the number of calories they are normally fed live one-third longer than those eating the usual diet. Caloric restriction also appears to improve memory and learning in laboratory rats. Several studies have demonstrated that rodents fed less over their lifetimes perform better in tests of cognitive function as they age and experience a delay in age-related memory loss.

Whether or not this is true in humans is unclear. It would be virtually impossible to control such an experiment. However, a study published in the *American Journal of Epidemiology* suggests that it may be true. Researchers at Loma Linda University began following ninety-nine healthy people in 1976, observing their dietary habits and caloric intake. Fifteen years later, when the study subjects were seventy-five years old, they were given tests that measured memory, language, and learning. It was found that those who ate more over the years scored lower on tests of cognitive function.

and many others promote a low-protein vegetarian diet. One diet book advises you to eat according to your blood type, while another recommends a Paleolithic (Stone Age) diet in which grains are avoided. There are programs that limit you to a few basic food choices, while others require a mathematics degree to figure out the portion sizes and proportions of the foods you should eat. It is no wonder people are confused!

What is the ideal diet? And more pointedly for readers of this book, what is the best diet for the preservation and improvement of memory and brain power? While I don't claim to be the diet guru of the Western world, I do know what the medical literature and scientific research say about these different diet philosophies. I've talked to—and even publicly debated—the originators and proponents of some of these divergent diets, and I understand their merits and their weaknesses. And for over twenty-five years

I've monitored thousands of patients on various diets. As a medical doctor, I've seen firsthand the powerful effects of food on the human body.

I want to tell you about the diet I recommend for the bulk of my patients. Of course, I make individual allowances for those with allergies, digestive problems, and even personal food preferences. Furthermore, variations in terms of portion size are an absolute must if excess weight is a factor. But I have found that the vast majority of the thousands and thousands of patients who have gone through my clinic do remarkably well on one common diet.

It's a diet most people can stick to. Unlike the extreme regimens that call for severe restriction of one food group—fats in some cases and carbohydrates in others—the diet I recommend is pretty "normal." There are no specific food items you have to eat in abundance. (Remember the grapefruit diet? The cabbage soup diet?) Nor do I put anything completely off limits forever. I believe that an occasional indulgence is good for the soul. As a result, because people have access to their own personal favorites among a variety of fresh, tasty, nutritious foods, compliance is high—and not just for two weeks or two months, which is how long most of us stay on "diets." In fact, I am loath to even call the food choices I recommend a "diet." The word itself smacks of deprivation and misery. Don't you get hungry just thinking about "going on a diet"?

Let's drop the word "diet." Instead, let's think of this as a lifelong nutrition guide or food plan. It's not about complicated food combinations or magic foods—although, as I will describe later in this chapter, there are a few foods that truly do merit the distinction of "brain foods." It's just about fresh, wholesome, largely unprocessed foods, foods close to the way nature made them— foods that our bodies were designed to eat.

## EAT TO RETARD AGING AND DEGENERATION

I recommend this food plan for people with memory deficits, neurological conditions, heart disease, hypertension, diabetes, cancer, arthritis, and almost all other medical conditions. Sometimes I am asked why I don't have specialized nutritional recommendations for each condition—a diabetic diet like the American Diabetes Association recommends, or a heart-healthy diet similar to the one espoused by the American Heart Association.

The reason is simple. As discussed in the previous chapter, there are specific mechanisms underlying *all* degenerative diseases and the aging process. Scientific studies have established firm relationships between these processes and degenerative disease. Let's review these mechanisms briefly.

- *Oxidation*, or *free-radical damage*, caused by normal metabolism and accelerated by environmental and lifestyle factors.

- *Glycation*, damage to proteins caused by their reaction with excess glucose.

- *Chronic inflammation*, resulting from an over-reactive immune system with release and lingering of harmful chemicals.

- *Defects in methylation*, the body's cellular housecleaning system, caused in part by inadequate levels of some of the B-complex vitamins.

Medical researchers have also demonstrated that the nutritional factors listed below can either accelerate or help control these destructive processes.

❑ Antioxidants prevent the destructive effects of free radicals. Some antioxidants are produced by your body, and others are obtained from the foods you eat (plant foods are the richest food sources of antioxidants) and from nutritional supplements (more on this in Step 2). On the other hand, certain foods, particularly fried foods and processed fats, are themselves sources of free radicals. And the more calories you consume, the more free radicals are produced.

❑ Disease states such as diabetes cause elevations in blood sugar (glucose) and increase the likelihood of glycation. So can diet, especially if it includes a high intake of sugar and refined carbohydrates that quickly break down into glucose.

❑ Certain fats known as essential fatty acids play an important role in inflammation. The types of fat you eat and take in supplement form can affect this process in a positive or negative way.

❑ Eating foods that are abundant in vitamins $B_6$, $B_{12}$, and folic acid will improve your body's methylation process. Supplementing these vitamins is even more important.

These are the guiding principles of my recommended food plan. This plan contains copious amounts of vegetables and fruits, along with legumes and whole grains, which are rich in antioxidants and B-complex vitamins. It's fairly high in carbohydrates, but not just any carbohydrates—fresh plant foods, yes;

## Foods High in Brain-Nourishing Nutrients

**Beta-Carotene**
Broccoli
Carrots
Cereal grass
Spinach
Sweet potatoes
Yellow squash

**Vitamin A**
Egg yolks
Fish liver oil
Green leafy
  vegetables

**Vitamin C**
Berries
Broccoli
Brussels sprouts
Citrus fruit
Green peppers

**Omega-3 Essential Fatty Acids**
Flaxseed
Flaxseed oil
Herring
Mackerel
Salmon
Sardines
Trout
Tuna

**Vitamin E**
Kale
Nuts
Olive oil
Pumpkin seeds
Sunflower seeds
Sweet potatoes
Wheat germ

**Folic Acid**
Asparagus
Brewer's yeast
Leafy greens
Legumes
Root vegetables

**Vitamin $B_6$**
Brussels sprouts
Cauliflower
Legumes
Nuts
Seeds
Whole grains

**Vitamin $B_{12}$**
Cheese
Eggs
Fish
Liver
Meat

refined flour and sugar, no. I suppose by fast-food standards these dietary recommendations would be considered relatively low in fat, but more important are the types of fats included —mainly unprocessed vegetable oils and fats from fish like salmon. The food plan also includes moderate amounts of protein from low-fat sources such as fish, legumes, and poultry.

Simple enough? It truly *is* simple, which is the beauty of this plan and why it is so easy to adhere to. Now that you understand the reasoning and medical underpinnings of this plan, I want to give you some specific guidelines and explain why these foods will nourish and protect your brain and improve your cognitive function.

## EAT PLENTY OF PROTECTIVE PLANT FOODS

The one food group you need to eat more of for better health is plant foods. Vegetables, fruits, whole grains, legumes, nuts, and seeds are truly the sustenance of life. Research has shown that the most powerful dietary measure you can take for improved health is to make vegetables and fruits the cornerstone of your diet. A plant-based diet lowers cholesterol, reduces the risk of heart disease, and strengthens bones. The risk of cancer is reduced twofold in people who eat larger than average amounts of plant foods. Vegetarians have a lower risk of heart disease and cancer than meat eaters do. They are also less likely to be overweight and, on average, live longer.

Plant foods are, for the most part, low in fat. And the fats these nutritious foods contain in their natural unprocessed state are the types of fat your body needs. Plants contain fiber, which improves digestion and reduces the risk of colon and breast cancer. Certain plants—whole grains, legumes, nuts and seeds, leafy greens, root vegetables, and cruciferous vegetables—are good sources of B-complex vitamins. (An exception is vitamin $B_{12}$, which is found only in meat and other animal-derived foods.) Plant foods are also nature's richest sources of antioxidant vitamins and minerals, which counteract oxidation, the number one contributor to aging and illness. Leafy green vegetables contain lots of vitamin A. Sweet potatoes, squash, and other yellow-orange vegetables are rich in beta-carotene. Unprocessed oils, whole grains, and raw nuts and seeds contain vitamin E. Citrus fruits, berries, and other fruits have high levels of vitamin C.

In addition, plant foods contain an abundance of *phytochemicals*. These are unique compounds produced by plants to protect them from environmental hazards, such as ultraviolet radiation from the sun, extremes of heat and cold, and insects. Although the study of phytochemicals is relatively new, we now know that many health-enhancing properties of plant foods come from these protective compounds. Scientists have only just begun to identify and catalogue individual phytochemicals, which will likely number in the tens of thousands. Of the hundreds discovered thus far, their actions are powerful and their names exotic. *Zeaxanthin* and *lutein,* found in leafy greens, protect the eyes. *Allicin* in garlic lowers cholesterol, protects the heart, and boosts the immune system. *Genistein* and *daidzein,* types of isoflavones found in soybeans, help balance hormones and defend against cancer. *Indoles* and *sulphoraphane* in broccoli detoxify carcinogens. Many phytochemicals also have potent antioxidant activity, including *proanthocyanidins* from grape seeds and *lycopene* from tomatoes.

Eating plant foods also may help prevent cognitive decline in your later years. A study published in 1998 in the *Journal of Neuroscience* found that certain fruits and vegetables actually improve memory. Researchers at the Human Nutrition Research Center on Aging at Tufts University in Boston, fed four groups of laboratory rats either a standard diet or a diet supplemented with one of the following—spinach, strawberry extract, or vitamin E. The spinach-fed rats had the best memories and fewest signs of nerve cell malfunction. This group was followed by the rats that had been fed strawberries, and then by the rats that had been supplemented with vitamin E. All three groups showed significant improvements over the rats that were fed the standard diet. The researchers concluded, ". . . phytochemicals present in antioxidant-rich foods, such as spinach, may be beneficial in retarding functional age-related central nervous system and cognitive behavioral deficits and, perhaps, may have some benefit in neurodegenerative disease."

# The Truth About Caffeine

Everybody "knows" that caffeine makes you more alert and clear-headed. Think again. A cup of coffee gives you a wakeup jolt because it triggers a stress response. Your adrenal glands are prompted to kick out the same stress hormones that are released when you perceive an external threat or danger. Your muscles tense, your blood sugar elevates for extra energy, your pulse and respiration rates speed up, and your state of alertness increases so you're ready to wrestle with or run from environmental dangers. You may be only sitting at your table or desk drinking a cup of coffee, but your body doesn't know that. It's preparing for action.

If you continue to drink coffee or other beverages containing caffeine throughout the day, your adrenal glands will be constantly stimulated and you will find yourself in a chronic state of stress. Extra stress, I guarantee, you don't need—it takes a toll on your body and brain. And even though most people think caffeine makes them mentally sharper, studies demonstrate that, in fact, the opposite is true.

Cut out caffeine, or at least strictly limit it to no more than one cup of coffee a day. A far better choice for a morning wakeup drink is green tea, which contains about a third of the caffeine of coffee and has proven health benefits. Be aware that colas and black tea are also significant sources of caffeine. (A more detailed discussion of how stress affects your memory and mental edge is presented in Step 7.)

## ALL CARBOHYDRATES ARE NOT CREATED EQUAL

Spinach, strawberries, beans, apples—all plant foods are made up primarily of carbohydrates. So are sodas, candy, sugar, and potato chips and most other snack foods. It's important that you understand the differences between various carbohydrate foods and how your body uses them.

Carbohydrates are your body's source of energy. When you eat a carbohydrate-containing food, enzymes in your gastrointestinal tract break it down into small sugar molecules (primarily glucose) that are absorbed into your bloodstream. In response to this rise in blood glucose, your pancreas releases *insulin,* a hormone that ushers glucose and other nutrients into the cells. Once in the cells, glucose is converted into energy. If immediate energy needs have been met, extra glucose may be converted to glycogen and stored in the liver and muscles for later use. Excess glucose may also be stored as fat.

You're probably familiar with the terms simple and complex carbohydrates. *Simple carbohydrates* are one- or-two-chain carbohydrates, which include most sugars. Longer-chain carbohydrates, like the starch and fiber of most vegetables and grains, are complex carbohydrates. We usually categorize processed grains like refined flour, which have had their fiber removed, as simple carbohydrates. As a rule, simple carbohydrates are quickly converted to glucose, causing a rapid elevation in blood sugar, followed by a sharp decline. Conversely, *complex carbohydrates* are broken down more slowly and result in a gradual, more sustained release of glucose. Ideally, our blood sugar should remain consistent—not too high and not too low—so we have a constant flow of energy. Therefore, complex carbohydrates, generally speaking, are preferable.

Although this simple-complex model has some value, nutritional research has moved beyond it. Researchers have found that some carbohydrates defy the simple-complex categorization. Some foods that we think of as complex—whole wheat bread, for example—actually break down and elevate blood sugar quite rapidly. And some "simple" carbohydrates, such as fruits, which consist mainly of a simple, one-molecule sugar called fructose, do not raise blood sugar as might be expected.

What has come out of this research is the *glycemic index* —a list of values assigned to foods that describe the rate at which blood glucose rises two or three hours after the foods are eaten. It is based on the blood glucose elevation caused by eating either glucose or white bread (the more recent indexes use white bread, as it is more typical of what we usually eat). The higher the glycemic index value of a given food, the faster and higher the blood sugar response. Many glycemic index values are predictable. Sodas and sweetened cereals are high; broccoli and beans are low. But many other foods might surprise you. For instance, ice cream and grapes are low, while potatoes and carrots are high. The glycemic index of common foods is presented in the inset on page 74. It is based on information from The Glycemic Research Institute.

You may be wondering how food and the glycemic index are related to memory and brain function. Well, like all of your body's tissues, your brain's preferred, almost exclusive, source of energy is glucose. Believe it or not, this small organ uses about 25 percent of your total glucose supplies. Because it functions twenty-four hours a day, the brain requires a constant source of energy. A slow, steady stream of glucose released into the bloodstream ensures a steady delivery of fuel to the brain, resulting in optimal brain functioning. However, low-glycemic carbohydrates, such as those listed on page 74, are quickly converted into glucose and enter the bloodstream in a rush, rapidly driving up glucose levels. Just as quickly, however, they fall, leaving a shortage of circulating glucose.

Although your brain has tremendous energy needs, it has few energy reserves. If glucose is not constantly supplied and the brain is unable to produce adequate energy, you may experience fatigue, mental confusion, irritability, and inability to focus. This extremely common occurrence is called *low blood sugar*, or *hypoglycemia*, and it was what Vivian, whose story I told you at the beginning of this chapter, suffered from. Most of us occasionally experience the "2:00 PM slump." An hour or two after a noontime meal of refined carbohydrates, your blood glucose falls sharply, leading to decreased brain energy production, fatigue, irritability, and difficulty in concentration.

Long-term overconsumption of high-glycemic carbohydrates wreaks havoc on the body's ability to properly regulate blood sugar. In addition to temporarily inducing low blood sugar levels, such dietary indiscretions are also associated with diabetes. Aging also throws in a monkey wrench. As we age, many of us experience a decreased ability to properly metabolize carbohydrates. The solution? Build your meals around low-glycemic carbohydrates. Most vegetables, fruits, and legumes prompt a slow release of glucose. By eating plant foods in their natural state, you won't have the high peaks and low valleys you get with refined carbohydrates. Energy, mood, and focus will remain steady.

One final comment on carbohydrates. As I stated before, one of the processes that contributes to aging and deterioration is glycation, which stems from the reaction of proteins with excess glucose. Unprocessed, low-glycemic carbohydrates will slow down this degenerative process and protect your body and brain from destructive AGEs.

## WE'RE ALL FATHEADS

Next time someone calls you a fathead, don't be offended. Your brain *is* more than 60-percent fat. Fats are an integral part of your brain's structure. The membranes of brain cells—of all cells, for that matter—are made up of fats. Fat is also a major component of myelin, the protective sheath that surrounds nerve axons and speeds up nerve conduction. In addition, fats affect the function of your brain. Certain fats are converted into powerful hormone-like substances called *prostaglandins* that have far-reaching effects in your body and brain. Yet, like carbohydrates, all fats are not created equal. Some are essential for health, while others are downright devastating.

Almost all foods contain fat, although some—animal products in particular—contain much more than others, such as fruits. The three major types of fat are saturated, unsaturated, and polyunsaturated.

*Saturated fats*, which are solid at room temperature, come from meat and dairy products, as well as tropical oils like palm and coconut. In spite of their bad reputation, saturated fats are not intrinsically bad. They are a component of cell membranes and a source of energy, insulation, and padding to protect your inner organs. Saturated fats do, however, tend to make platelets in the blood stick together, and they can build up in arteries and organs. This contributes to both obesity and heart disease. Your body is able to manufacture all the saturated fats it needs, so you don't really need to eat any saturated fat at all. Eating a little is fine, but the typical American eats far too much saturated fat. Perhaps more important, we eat saturated fats at the expense of

## Glycemic Index of Common Foods

### White Bread = 100

*The following list is limited to carbohydrate-containing foods. Foods that contain mostly fat or protein do not cause blood sugar levels to rise significantly.*

### Low-Glycemic Foods (fine to eat in abundance)

- All fresh and frozen fruits, except for dried fruits, most tropical fruits, and most melons (see high-glycemic foods listed below for exceptions).

- All fresh and frozen vegetables, except for corn and most root vegetables (see list of high-glycemic foods listed below for exceptions).

- All beans, peas, and legumes (dried and fresh varieties are better than canned).

- Selected breads (sprouted grain, whole grain rye, and whole wheat tortillas).

- Selected cereals (bran, slow-cooking oatmeal).

- Pasta (except for gnocchi that is made from potatoes).

- Whole grains (pearled barley, rye, wheat kernels, couscous, and bulgur).

- Dairy products (milk, yogurt, cottage cheese, cheese—low-fat versions are healthiest).

- Soy milk.

- Selected snack foods in moderation (graham crackers, sponge cake).

certain unsaturated fats that our bodies cannot manufacture—fats that are absolutely essential for optimal health.

There are two types of *unsaturated fats,* monounsaturated and polyunsaturated. There is a common belief that *monounsaturated fats,* like olive, canola, peanut, and almond oil, are the healthiest fats. Not so. It isn't that these monounsaturated oils are un-

- Salsa, mustard, and ketchup in small amounts.
- Fructose (not high-fructose corn syrup), brown rice syrup, xylitol, and stevia.

### High-Glycemic Foods (avoid or eat sparingly)

- Dried fruits (dried apricots are acceptable in moderation).
- Fruit juices (if you must have juice, limit it to 4 ounces of unsweetened apple, grapefruit, orange, peach, pear, or pineapple juice).
- Tropical fruits (pineapples, mangos, ripe bananas, papayas, and kiwis).
- Sweetened applesauce.
- Watermelon, cantaloupe, and casaba melon.
- Corn.
- Root vegetables (beets, parsnips, turnips, and potatoes—best are new red potatoes. Yams and sweet potatoes are acceptable).
- Most breads (white, whole wheat, sourdough, and bagels).
- Most cereals (most cold cereals, instant oatmeal, and Cream of Wheat or Rice).
- Rice (long-grain brown rice and brown Basmati rice are best, but should be eaten in moderation).
- Most snack foods (chips, rice cakes, popcorn, pretzels, cookies, and candy).
- Sucrose (white sugar), corn syrup, honey, maple syrup, and molasses.

healthy. They too are a part of the structure of our cell membranes, and they protect against heart disease by keeping our arteries flexible. This is one reason they've earned their popular reputation as healthy fats. However, they do not have the biological activity of the polyunsaturated fats we'll discuss below. One of the best qualities of monounsaturated fats is that they are relatively stable. Unlike polyunsaturated fats, they don't break down into harmful components when heated. (See the discussion of trans fatty acids on page 77.) Monounsaturated oils are fine in moderation but, again, they aren't essential—your body is able to produce them. I highly recommend olive oil for cooking, but it shouldn't be used exclusively in place of more important polyunsaturated fats.

The most important dietary fats are *polyunsaturated fats,* which are found in vegetable oils, nuts and seeds, and cold-water fish. They are the most biologically active of all fats and are involved in energy production, cellular membrane structure, and a host of other functions. Within this class of fats are two unique nutrients known as *essential fatty acids (EFAs),* which play vital roles in the maintenance of health and the optimal functioning of the brain. (We will discuss EFAs and "brain fats" in detail in Step 4.)

There are two important facts you need to know about EFAs in this discussion on diet. First, the body cannot manufacture EFAs—they must come from dietary or supplement sources. Second, it is important that the two types of EFAs be eaten in balance. The EFAs are grouped into two classes, based on their chemical structures: *omega-3* and *omega-6 fatty acids.* The primary dietary sources of omega-6 fatty acids are vegetable oils, which we eat in abundance. The primary sources of omega-3 fatty acids are cold-water fish like salmon, mackerel, and sardines, and flaxseed oil, which most of us eat in small quantities, if at all. As a result, our diets typically are precariously tilted towards omega-6s. According to Dr. Michael A. Schmidt, author of *Smart Fats,* the ideal ratio of dietary omega-6 to omega-3 fatty acids is 1:1—and certainly no more than 4:1—while the average American's current ratio is 20:1 or 30:1.

Make it a point to increase your consumption of omega-3 fatty acids. Eat salmon and other cold-water fish several times a week. Use flaxseed oil for salad dressings and other recipes that do not require the oil to be heated. You can also grind fresh, whole flaxseeds in a coffee grinder and sprinkle them on salads and cereals, or drink it in juice or a smoothie. And when you eat vegetable oils and nut butters, make sure they're in their natural state. Omega-3 and omega-6 fatty acids are very fragile. Exposure to heat, light, even oxygen triggers oxidative damage to these oils and produces free radicals. As discussed earlier, free radicals contribute to brain dysfunction, as well as overall health degeneration.

Purchase only unrefined, organic vegetable oils and raw nut butters—you'll find them in your health food store—and store them in the refrigerator. Avoid foods that have been fried in vegetable oils. Also, stay away from products made with hydrogenated or partially hydrogenated vegetable oils. This includes items such as margarine, commercial baked goods, and many prepared foods. These vegetable oils have been subjected to heat and chemical processes to extend shelf life and make them solid at room temperature. This process reconfigures their chemical structure, creating harmful substances called *trans fatty acids.* In fact, any time a vegetable oil is heated to high temperatures (think French fries and other fried foods) trans fatty acids are likely produced. These unnatural fats have no nutritional value, and they have been linked to cancer, diabetes, infertility, obesity, and low birth weight, and, according to Dr. Walter Willet of Harvard's School of Public Health, they may be responsible for 30,000 deaths a year!

### PROTEIN POWER

Proteins make up the majority of our tissues. They are essential for growth and tissue repair and act as a carrier of important components in the blood. During digestion, proteins are broken down into amino acids. This makes them very important to the brain because many neurotransmitters are made of amino acids. In fact, some amino acids act as neurotransmitters.

The problem with protein is that it is most concentrated in high-fat meat, eggs, and dairy products. However, there are lower-fat sources, such as skinless poultry, fish, egg whites, low-fat and fat-free dairy products, tofu, beans and legumes, and whole grains. While it is important to eat some protein at every meal, many of us get too much. Excess protein has a downside. It's hard on the kidneys, and years of overeating protein can contribute to osteoporosis or thinning of the bones in older age. Most important, a fatty acid found in meat, dairy products, and eggs, called *arachidonic acid,* is one of the principal fats in your brain. When it is out of balance with other fatty acids, arachidonic acid can form highly inflammatory and sometimes damaging prostaglandins.

Three to four small servings of protein-rich foods per day will supply you with all the protein you need. A serving size of animal protein is about the size of a deck of cards; a serving of plant protein is the size of a tennis ball. (Compare that to the monster servings you got the last time you ate in a restaurant.) Even if you're eating a primarily vegetarian diet, as long as you include some eggs, low-fat or nonfat dairy, whole grains, and beans and legumes, you will get plenty of protein.

## BEWARE OF FOOD ADDITIVES

At last count, over 3,000 chemicals are added to our food to improve taste and appearance and to retard spoilage. I am particularly concerned about the effects of two widely used food additives—monosodium glutamate and aspartame. They are both toxic to the brain.

### Monosodium Glutamate

Monosodium glutamate (MSG) is a very powerful taste enhancer. Food manufacturers love it because it perks up the flavor of the blandest of foods. Tons of it are added to our food supply every year. MSG contains the amino acid glutamate. As discussed in Chapter 2, glutamate is one of the brain's most common chemical messengers, or neurotransmitters. Although many neurotransmitters use amino acids as building blocks, glutamate is used by the brain in its unaltered state. Glutamate is known as an *excitatory neurotransmitter* because it activates neurons and causes them to fire repeatedly. Under normal circumstances, this activity is balanced by calming inhibitory neurotransmitters, and excess glutamate is cleared away. However, when you ingest MSG, it's like mainlining glutamate—it simply overwhelms your brain.

According to neurosurgeon Russell Blaylock, M.D., author of *Excitotoxins, the Taste That Kills,* excess glutamate literally excites neurons to death—they run out of energy, degenerate, and die. People who are especially sensitive to MSG have reactions every time they eat it. However, in large enough doses, MSG is neurotoxic to everyone, and it is especially detrimental to young, developing brains.

Read food labels carefully. MSG is particularly well disguised and is present in a number of additives, including hydrolyzed vegetable protein, yeast extract, seasonings, natural flavorings, stock, broth, and bouillon.

## Asparatame

Aspartame (NutraSweet) is the most popular artificial sweetener on the market, and it is present in over 5,000 foods and drinks. It is a mixture of two amino acids—aspartate and phenylalanine. Like glutamate, aspartate acts as an excitatory neurotransmitter in its unaltered state. And high concentrations of aspartate can overexcite and damage neurons. In addition, NutraSweet is further broken down into methanol (wood alcohol) and other toxic chemicals that are known to have a negative effect on the brain, even causing brain tumors in some cases. Thousands of adverse reactions to aspartame have been reported to the FDA over the years, but they have been largely ignored. Many of these reactions—dizziness, mood changes, vision problems, headaches, and even seizures—involve the brain and central nervous system.

## TIPS FOR IMPLEMENTING A BRAIN-HEALTHY FOOD PLAN

The food plan presented in this chapter is relatively easy to follow, but it will take a conscientious effort. Our fast-paced lifestyles are convenience oriented. It's so easy to pick up some fast food, call for a pizza delivery, or head for a restaurant. Defrosting a frozen entrée is certainly easier than preparing a dinner of healthy whole foods yourself. However, the payoffs of eating healthy are enormous. In the long run you'll enjoy a trimmer body, a healthier heart, better controlled blood sugar, improved overall health, and a clearer mind. Here are some tips to make implementing this food plan easier.

## Carbohydrates

- Make vegetables the focus of your meals. Eat five to eight servings of vegetables every day (1 serving = 1 cup raw or $1/2$ cup cooked). Limit high-glycemic vegetables such as corn and potatoes to twice a week.

- Eat three or four servings of fruit daily (1 serving = 1 medium whole fruit or $1/2$ cup sliced).

- Limit grain-based foods to three or four servings per day (1 serving = 1 cup cooked whole grains, whole-grain cereals or pasta, or 1 slice bread). Go easy on bread. Most of us eat too much of the wrong kinds. The only kinds of breads I recommend are whole-grain rye and sprouted grain breads, which have a much lower glycemic index than any other bread, including whole-wheat breads.

- Become familiar with the glycemic index of foods you like, and eat mostly those foods that cause a slow release of blood sugar. Avoid sugary foods, most baked goods, cold cereals, white rice, and other refined grains. (See the Glycemic Index Chart on page 74.)

## Fat

- Eat cold-water fish like salmon, mackerel, herring, sardines, tuna, and trout, which contain brain-boosting omega-3 essential fatty acids, several times a week.

- Avoid processed foods made with fat. This includes most baked goods, peanut butter, and prepared frozen meals. Buy raw, organic nut butters and unrefined, cold-processed, expeller-pressed oils. You'll find these in your local health food store. Store these products in the refrigerator.

- Do not eat margarine, which contains dangerous trans fatty acids. Instead, use a drizzle of olive oil.

- Incorporate omega-3-rich flaxseed into your diet. Use 1 to 3 table-spoons of flaxseed oil or $1/4$ cup freshly ground seeds every day. (Never heat flaxseed oil.) Sprinkle the seeds on a salad or cereal, or mix them into a drink. For a flaxseed oil salad dressing, mix the following ingredients together:

*2 tablespoons flaxseed oil*
*1 tablespoon lemon juice or vinegar (balsamic is particularly good)*
*1 clove crushed garlic*
*Salt (or low-sodium seasoning) and pepper to taste*

## Protein

- Several times a week, make your main protein source brain-healthy cold-water fish, such as salmon, mackerel, herring, sardines, tuna, and trout. (1 serving = 4 to 6 ounces.)

- Relegate meat and poultry to side-dish status. (1 serving = 4 to 6 ounces.)

- Eat protein-rich plant foods, such as beans (1 serving = $1/2$ cup cooked), raw nuts and seeds (1 serving = 4 tablespoons nuts/seeds, or 2 tablespoons nut butter), tofu (1 serving = 4 to 6 ounces), nonfat or lowfat yogurt or cottage cheese (1 serving = 1 cup), and soy milk (1 serving = 1 cup).

- Eggs are a good protein source, and recent research indicates that they do not raise cholesterol in a majority of people. They also contain DHA, an important brain fat, and choline, a B-vitamin relative that is important for brain health. (1 serving = 2 eggs or 1 egg yolk mixed with 3 egg whites.)

## Miscellaneous

- Drink plenty of filtered or purified water—8 to 12 eight-ounce glasses per day. Avoid tap water.

- Avoid MSG and aspartame (NutraSweet). Read labels carefully, as these harmful additives are added to thousands and thousands of foods.

## SUMMING IT UP

Some 2,400 years ago, when Hippocrates said, "Let food be thy medicine," he was really onto something. We now know why food has such a huge impact on our health and mental function. By incorporating the sound dietary principles presented in Step 1, you will take a giant step toward improved memory and mental edge.

For those of you who already eat healthy foods, these dietary recommendations will be easy to adapt. For others, this food plan may present more of a challenge. If you fall into this category, my advice is simple: Go at your own pace. If you cannot clean up your diet overnight, don't worry about it. Just begin by taking a few steps at a time in the right direction. Eventually, you'll end up where you want to be. Persistence is the key.

As important as diet is, I strongly believe that it is virtually impossible for you to get all of the vitamins, minerals, and other nutrients your body needs from diet alone. In Step 2, you will discover the importance of nutrient supplementation for optimal health and brain function.

$$\text{STEP } 2$$

# Protect Your Brain
# With Vitamins and Minerals

*Sally was seventy-two years old when I first met her. She was suffer-ing from such severe memory loss and depression that her family had been advised to place her in a nursing home. Her daughter brought her to my office in a last-ditch effort to see if anything else could be done. Sally was lethargic, and her answers to my questions were brief and incomplete. She could not give the correct year or name the president of the United States—commonly asked questions to determine a patient's mental state.*

*I placed Sally on a nutritional supplement program consisting of high doses of antioxidants with extra vitamin E, B-complex vitamins, essential fatty acids, and other nutrients that target the brain. I also gave her a vitamin $B_{12}$ injection and continued giving her twice-a-week injections for the next month.*

*When Sally and her daughter returned a month later, I looked into the eyes of a different woman. She was alert, smiling, and made pleas-ant small talk. Her daughter said that her mother's mood and memory were so much improved that they were no longer considering a nursing home. I did nothing heroic in Sally's care. I simply identified and treat-ed underlying nutritional deficiencies.*

I have been practicing medicine for over twenty-five years. After graduating from medical school, I completed a medical-surgical internship and began a residency in orthopedic surgery. As my horizons expanded beyond the cloistered walls of medical school, I discovered remarkable healing tools and techniques that weren't being taught in medical school or used in hospitals. I met individuals like Nathan Pritikin, who had developed a low-fat nutritional program to treat patients with serious heart disease when drugs and surgery failed. I discovered the work of two-time Nobel Prize winner Dr. Linus Pauling on vitamin C, and the research of other nutritional pioneers. I also met and learned from physicians like Dr. William Currier, who had actually given up a conventional medical practice to specialize in nutritional medicine.

As I spoke to my colleagues at the hospital about these remarkable nutritional therapies, I was astounded at their indifference. If the treatment being discussed wasn't a surgical procedure or a pharmaceutical drug, nobody wanted to hear about it. Although I loved medicine, I was having serious doubts about the medical profession, and especially about its reluctance to consider innovative therapies that would obviously help many patients.

At that point I decided to choose the path less traveled. I began a serious study of the medical literature on nutrition and educated myself on the use of diet and vitamin and mineral supplementation. I worked for a time at Dr. Currier's and Nathan Pritikin's clinics so I could soak up their experience and knowledge. In 1979, I opened the Whitaker Wellness Institute and began using diet, exercise, and nutritional supplements as the primary therapies to treat serious diseases. With these simple "low-tech" therapies, hundreds of heart patients have successfully avoided bypass surgery. Patients with diabetes and hypertension have augmented their conventional treatments with this nutritional approach. And thousands of patients with all manners of disease have been able to replace their medications with far safer natural therapies.

I share this story of my evolution into nutritional medicine because I want you to understand where I'm coming from. Nutritional supplementation is a very important part of my medical practice. When I first opened Whitaker Wellness Institute over twenty years ago, I assumed that diet and exercise were the most important healing tools. With the passing years, however, I have become convinced that nutritional supplements are equally, if not more, important. In this step of the program, I'm going to present the most basic and, for the sake of prevention, the most important natural brain protectors—vitamins and minerals.

# Aging and Nutritional Supplements

From birth to age twenty-five, you're getting better and better. Age twenty-five is considered the apex of health in the human species—never again will your reflexes be as sharp, your eyesight as keen, your muscles as powerful, your bones as dense, your heart and lungs as strong, or your organ systems as efficient. After age twenty-five, however, the body begins a downslide. It's slow and gentle at first, then it begins picking up more and more momentum as one approaches age fifty. After that, the slide really hits the floorboard. Physiologically, there's a lot of difference between a healthy twenty-five-year-old and a healthy fifty-year-old. But the difference between a healthy fifty-year-old and a healthy seventy-five-year-old is enormous. The pace of physical decline just keeps on speeding up as the effects of the aging process accumulate.

In my opinion, the most important thing you can do to slow down this inevitable degeneration is to bathe your cells in nutrients—the raw materials it needs to function at its best. Feed it copious amounts of antioxidant vitamins and minerals to fight free radicals. Supply it with B-complex vitamins to facilitate the methylation process. Strengthen your bones with calcium, your heart with coenzyme $Q_{10}$, and your cell membranes with essential fatty acids. Improve your circulation with *Ginkgo biloba*. Not only does your body's production of these important nutrients decline with age, your requirements for them increase.

Nutritional supplementation is good for kids (I give my young children vitamins and minerals every day). It is important for young adults. But it is absolutely vital for anyone over fifty.

## SUPPLEMENTATION AND OPTIMAL NUTRITION

A food plan to enhance brain function and overall health was presented in Step 1, but the best of food plans will benefit you only if you follow it. Unfortunately, very few Americans come even close to eating a decent diet. Only 9 percent of Americans eat the recommended five daily servings of plant foods. And according to a U.S. Department of Agriculture (USDA) survey of 11,658 Americans, on an average day, 41 percent eat no fruit at all, 72 percent eat no vitamin-C rich fruits, 82 percent eat no cruciferous vegetables such as broccoli and cabbage, and 84 percent eat no high-fiber, whole-grain foods. These folks (and statistically speaking, you're likely to be among them) are headed toward trouble—if not now, then as they get older when their body's internal production of protective nutrients declines. The only way they are going to get the vitamins and minerals they need is by taking nutritional supplements.

In addition, over 70 percent of the food the average American eats has been processed. As explained in Step 1, processed foods are stripped of fiber. Their natural, health-enhancing fats and oils are damaged by heat and chemicals, creating free radicals and harmful trans fatty acids. And the vitamin, mineral, and phyto-chemical content of processed foods is significantly reduced.

Even if you are among the small minority who eat right, I am firmly convinced that it is simply naive to assume you can get optimal nutrition from diet alone. The nutrient content of plant foods depends upon the quality of the soil in which crops are grown. The soils of certain areas of the world are naturally defi-cient in certain minerals, and foods grown in those soils are low in those particular nutrients. For example, the cancer rate in var-ious areas of China varies by a factor of three. These differences have been traced to the small amount of selenium, a mineral that reduces the risk of cancer, in the soils of these areas. People living in low-selenium areas (and presumably eating food grown in these mineral-poor soils) are three times more likely to get cancer than their countrymen living in high-selenium areas. Sure, farm-ers add minerals to the soil in the form of fertilizers, but econom-ics dictates that they replace only the few minerals that ensure crop growth. Other minerals, which are important in small amounts for optimal health, are ignored.

Storage is another nutrient killer. Once plant foods have been harvested, their nutritional value begins to drop. The longer they are stored, the more significant the nutrient losses. You may be surprised to learn that certain fruits and vegetables—apples, potatoes, and other root vegetables, for example—can be stored for months on end. Freezing produce tends to lock in nutrients, but whether or not these nutrients remain intact depends on how the frozen items are handled during shipping and storage. Every time a frozen food even partially defrosts and is refrozen, nutrients are lost.

Based on all of these factors, I firmly believe that every man, woman, and child should take a multivitamin and mineral supplement every day. If nothing else, think of it as "health insurance" against the inadequacies of our modern-day diets. Supplementation becomes especially important as we get older. Our digestive systems aren't as efficient as they used to be, and our ability to extract nutrients from food becomes compromised. The resulting nutritional deficiencies jeopardize all aspects of our health—and brain function is no exception.

Researchers at the USDA mounted a study to examine how nutritional deficiencies affect memory and mental function. They determined the nutritional status of twenty-eight healthy people age sixty and older, and then gave them challenging mental tasks to measure cognitive function. Significant relationships were noted between nutritional status and test performance. Subjects who had optimal levels of certain nutrients tested better than those with nutrient deficiencies. Their EEG readings, which measure electrical activity in the brain, indicated better brain functioning. This study suggested that even mild nutritional deficits might be responsible for mental slowdowns and changes in brain function. The strongest associations were with thiamin (vitamin $B_1$), riboflavin (vitamin $B_2$), and iron. Beta-carotene, vitamin C, and zinc levels were also predictive of performance on mental function tests.

A larger, longer term study carried out at the University of New Mexico School of Medicine followed 137 people between age sixty-six and ninety for six years. The participants in this study were educated, well nourished, and had no memory problems. Their vitamin status was determined at the beginning of the study and again after six years. At the study's conclusion they were given tests of cognitive function. Test performance was related to past and current nutritional status, and significant associations between mental function and vitamin status were noted. Those in the study group who had higher blood levels and intake of vitamins in the B-complex family—thiamin, riboflavin, niacin, and folate—performed better in tests of abstract thinking. High blood levels of vitamin C were associated with increased ability in performing visual and spatial tasks, and higher intake of vitamins E, A, $B_6$, and $B_{12}$ correlated with better scores on visual and spatial recall and/or abstract thinking. The participants in this study who, on their own, had taken vitamin supplements, did better on difficult visual and spatial tests and on tests of abstract thinking.

As these studies make clear, supplementing your diet with essential vitamins and minerals is an absolute must if you are interested in slowing down the aging process and sustaining optimal function. Let's look at the individual nutrients that have been identified as having important roles in brain health. Table 4.1 on page 100, presents a listing of these nutrients as well as their recommended daily dosages.

## B-Complex Vitamins

Among the most important nutrients in maintaining optimal mental functioning are the B-complex vitamins. As explained in previous chapters, the importance of the B vitamins has been underscored by new research on methylation—the process by which toxic byproducts of cellular metabolism are removed from the body. When this process goes awry, there is a buildup of highly toxic *homocysteine.* Elevated homocysteine is a known contributor to atherosclerosis and has been classified as an independent risk factor for heart disease and stroke.

In recent years, excess homocysteine has also been linked to neurodegenerative disorders. In addition to damaging blood vessels in the brain and decreasing blood flow and, thus, nutrient and oxygen delivery to brain cells, homocysteine also appears to damage certain receptor sites in the brain. High levels of homocysteine are a marker for memory loss and cognitive dysfunction. In a study carried out at the Human Nutrition Research Center on Aging at Tufts University, a strong association was noted between homocysteine levels, vascular disease, and performance on tests of cognitive function. The patients with the highest levels of homocysteine and vascular disease scored lowest on tests of cognitive function.

There is also a link between elevated homocysteine levels and Alzheimer's disease. Researchers at the University of Oxford in Great Britain, measured the homocysteine levels of 164 patients over age fifty-five who had been diagnosed with Alzheimer's. These levels were compared to those of 108 people in the same age group who had normal mental function. The researchers found that Alzheimer's disease was 4.5 times more common in the people with the highest homocysteine levels. They also discovered that levels of vitamin $B_{12}$ and folic acid, the primary B vitamins involved in methylation (vitamin $B_6$ plays a supporting role), were considerably lower in the patients with Alzheimer's. Those with the lowest levels of vitamin $B_{12}$ and folic acid were 4.3 and 3.3 times, respectively, more likely to have Alzheimer's than people with the highest levels of these nutrients.

In addition to facilitating methylation and helping control homocysteine levels, several members of the B-complex family of vitamins serve independent protective functions in the brain. Supplementation with these nutrients is especially important as we grow older, because while full-blown deficiencies of these B vitamins are rare, subtle deficiencies are quite common. When supplementing with B-complex vitamins, don't single out one or two—take the whole family. They work best together; deficiencies in one or another may upset the teamwork.

### Choline

Classified by the National Academy of Sciences as an essential nutrient in 1998, choline falls into the general category of B-complex vitamins. It is a constituent of cell membranes and a precursor of the neurotransmitter acetylcholine, which is important in memory and learning. Choline is especially important for the developing brain, and studies have demonstrated that the offspring of laboratory animals that were denied adequate choline during pregnancy scored poorly on tests of attention span and memory. Other studies showed that these offspring continued to have cognitive deficits throughout their lives. The protective effect of prenatal choline even extended into old age, as animals whose mothers received supplemental choline bypassed normal age-related memory declines. According to Dr. Christina Williams of Duke University, one of the scientists involved in these studies, ". . . supplementation with choline during the last third of pregnancy has fairly dramatic and long-lasting effects on the memory of offspring."

Because choline is an important part of the fatty membranes of brain cells, it will be addressed again in Step 4, "Nourish Your Brain With Fats."

SUGGESTED DOSAGE: *425 milligrams of choline daily for the general population, 450 milligrams for pregnant women, and 550 milligrams for nursing mothers.*

## Folic Acid

Supplemental folic acid is important for men and women of all ages. Deficiencies are associated with irritability, paranoia, and memory loss. In addition to its very specific role in the methylation process, folic acid is required for DNA synthesis. It is necessary for proper cell division and for the development of the nervous system in the fetus. For this reason, folic acid supplementation is vital for all women of childbearing age. Folic acid deficiencies during pregnancy are linked with birth defects of the neural tube, such as spina bifida.

SUGGESTED DOSAGE: *400 micrograms of folic acid daily. Folate, the form of folic acid found in food, is poorly absorbed, so supplementation of this vitamin is essential.*

## Vitamin B$_1$ (Thiamin)

Vitamin B$_1$, also known as thiamin, was the first of the B vitamins to be discovered. It is required in the production of three important enzymes that are necessary for the conversion of glucose into energy in the brain. This nutrient also mimics the activities of the important neurotransmitter acetylcholine. Extreme deficiencies in thiamin cause a condition known as beriberi, which is characterized by mental confusion and other symptoms.

Thiamin supplementation appears to improve cognitive function. In a study spearheaded by David Benton at the University of Wales, 120 young women were administered 50 milligrams of either thiamin or a placebo every day for two months. Tests measuring the subjects' mood, memory, and reaction times were given at the start of the study and repeated at its conclusion. Although memory, per se, did not improve with thiamin supplementation, the women taking the thiamin supplements felt more clearheaded, composed, and energetic. Their reaction times were faster as well. It is important to note that none of these women had what would be considered low thiamin status at the study's onset—they were all measured in the normal range.

**Suggested Dosage:** *50 milligrams of vitamin $B_1$ daily. (Higher therapeutic doses of 3 to 8 grams have been used in the treatment of Alzheimer's disease with positive results and little or no adverse side effects.)*

### *Vitamin $B_3$ (Niacin)*

Vitamin $B_3$ is necessary for the production of energy. Its principal supplemental use is for the lowering of cholesterol. In the brain, niacin is located both in the nerve cell membranes, where it helps facilitate impulse transmission, and inside brain cells, where it is involved in metabolism and oxygen supply. A number of studies have shown that supplementing various forms of this nutrient improves brain function. In one such study, published in the journal *Psychopharmacology*, forty-three participants, ranging in age from thirty-five to eighty-five, were tested for short- and long-term memory. They were given either vitamin $B_3$ (in a form containing 141.7 milligrams of nicotinic acid) or a placebo. When the memory tests were repeated after eight weeks of supplementation, test results revealed 10- to 40-percent improvements in both short-term and long-term memory, compared to the placebo group.

Deficiencies in vitamin $B_3$ have been linked to short-term memory loss, fatigue, depression, and dementia. Vitamin $B_3$ has been used as a treatment for mental disorders, such as schizophrenia.

**Suggested Dosage:** *100 milligrams of vitamin $B_3$ daily. Do not take the time-release form of niacin, as it may cause liver damage.*

### Vitamin $B_5$ (Pantothenic Acid)

Vitamin $B_5$ is required in energy production. It is also involved in the synthesis of adrenal hormones and red blood cells. Vitamin $B_5$'s greatest benefits for the brain are derived from its role in the synthesis of the neurotransmitter acetylcholine, which is involved in memory and learning. Without adequate supplies of pantothenic acid, your body cannot convert choline into acetylcholine.

SUGGESTED DOSAGE: *50 milligrams of vitamin $B_5$ daily.*

### Vitamin $B_6$ (Pyridoxine)

Vitamin $B_6$, also known as pyridoxine, is necessary for the formation of red blood cells, structural proteins, and prostaglandins. It plays a supporting role in methylation and is required in the production of some of the brain's neurotransmitters—norepinephrine, serotonin, and dopamine. It has been shown to enhance memory and brain function in older individuals, and low levels of this nutrient correspond to poor scores on tests of cognitive function. Vitamin $B_6$ deficiencies are not uncommon in the aging population.

SUGGESTED DOSAGE: *75 milligrams of vitamin $B_6$ daily.*

### Vitamin $B_{12}$ (Cobalamin)

Also known as cobalamin, vitamin $B_{12}$ is the most important of the B vitamins for proper brain functioning. In addition to its role in the methylation process, vitamin $B_{12}$ is involved in the production of red blood cells, as well as the myelin sheaths that cover and protect neurons and help speed up impulse conduction. Deficiencies of vitamin $B_{12}$ are common in the elderly and may result in mental confusion that is sometimes mistaken for Alzheimer's disease. In fact, $B_{12}$ deficiency is a primary cause of reversible dementia and is responsible for as much as one-third of the mental deterioration and confusion in older people. Although estimates vary, one study found that 42 percent of people over sixty-five had a $B_{12}$ deficiency.

Even if we get adequate amounts of this vitamin from eating meat, fish, eggs, and cheese, aging often reduces our ability to absorb it. This is because of an age-related decline in the production of stomach acid, as well as a substance called *intrinsic factor*, both of which are required for the absorption of vitamin $B_{12}$.

Extreme $B_{12}$ deficiencies may cause pernicious anemia, a very serious form of anemia that is associated with nerve damage. Many physicians, however, tend to overlook the possibility of a $B_{12}$ deficiency if pernicious anemia is not present. They may forget that memory loss and other mental declines may be signs of a less severe $B_{12}$ deficiency. Testing serum homocysteine, serum cobalamin, or urinary methylmalonic acid may pick up these more modest deficiencies. These tests, which can be done in a physician's office, give a more reliable reading of true vitamin $B_{12}$ reserves.

Vitamin $B_{12}$ deficiencies can be remedied by injections of 1,000 micrograms of this vitamin. In one study, injections completely reversed the mental deficits of 61 percent of older patients with low vitamin $B_{12}$ levels. The remaining 39 percent of the people in the study may have had long-term vitamin deficiencies that could not be treated by supplementation. Patients who have had symptoms for less than one year respond the best to $B_{12}$ supplementation. This underscores the importance of paying attention to changes in your mental function and in those of your loved ones.

Be sure to request the tests mentioned above if you begin to notice declines. But be aware that even massive doses of vitamin $B_{12}$ cannot change the course of more serious forms of cognitive dysfunction, such as Alzheimer's disease. The 10-step program described in this book is designed to prevent memory loss and treat it in its earliest stages when it is still reversible.

SUGGESTED DOSAGE: *I start my patients on injections of 1,000 micrograms of vitamin $B_{12}$ twice a week for one month to replenish supplies in the liver. Shots are administered twice a month after that. (I usually teach the patient or a family member how to administer the injections at home.) I recommend to all of my patients—even those without symptoms—to begin these injections around age sixty. Vitamin $B_{12}$ injections not only improve memory but lift mood, as well.*

*For those who do not want injections, 1,000 micrograms of vitamin*

$B_{12}$ *in sublingual doses, which are dissolved under the tongue, usually suffice. However, for more serious memory impairment, I highly recommend the injections.*

*For younger, healthier individuals, I suggest a daily oral dose of 100 micrograms of vitamin $B_{12}$.*

## Antioxidants

Free radicals, as explained in Chapter 3, are unstable, highly reactive atoms or molecules that are byproducts of normal metabolism. To stabilize themselves, free radicals steal electrons from atoms and molecules they come into contact with, destabilizing them and turning them into free radicals. Thus, a self-perpetuating chain reaction of free radical or oxidative damage is set in motion. Enter antioxidants. Your body produces a multitude of antioxidants—lipoic acid, superoxide dismutase (SOD), glutathione, to name a few. Your diet also supplies you with antioxidants, as discussed in Step 1 of the program. Antioxidants stabilize free radicals by giving them an electron and breaking the destructive cycle. Without antioxidants we would literally be eaten up by free radicals.

However, despite the protective actions of antioxidants, oxidative damage accumulates slowly and systemically throughout the body over the years, and your brain is not spared. In fact, because of its high fat content and high consumption of oxygen, the brain is exceptionally vulnerable to the ravages of oxidation. Free-radical damage has been identified in the brain's frontal and temporal lobes—areas involved in learning and memory.

So you see how important antioxidants are to the health and smooth functioning of your brain. Making sure your body is supplied with an abundance of these nutrients is vital for optimal health. The older you get, the fewer antioxidants your body is able to produce. At the same time, your need for them increases. Of course, if you eat fruits, vegetables, legumes, raw nuts, whole grains, and unprocessed oils, you'll get some of these crucial nutrients from your diet. But all things considered, supplementing with a broad array of antioxidant vitamins is your best means of defending against oxidative stress to the brain and other tis-

## How Keen Are Your Powers of Observation?

With so many stimuli competing for your attention, your brain is constantly filtering out information that is not worth remembering. The following quiz evaluates your observations of everyday items. It shows how your mind neglects to store nonessential information. During the quiz, you'll probably find yourself saying, "I should know that!"

1. Whose picture is on a twenty-dollar bill? What is pictured on the back of the bill?

2. On which side of a woman's blouse are the buttons?

3. Is the red light on the top or bottom of a traffic light?

4. Which continent is larger, South America or Africa?

5. On which side of the phone is the star symbol (*)?

6. What shape is a yield sign?

7. How many keys are on your key ring?

8. What color is the top stripe on an American flag?

9. What color are your best friend's eyes?

10. On a phone, what number is represented by the letters ABC?

*Answers: 1. Andrew Jackson is on the front; the White House is on the back. 2. The left side. 3. The top. 4. Africa. 5. The left. 6. An upside-down triangle. 8. Red. 10. The number 2 button.*

sues. Let's look at vitamins E, C, A and beta-carotene—the most important antioxidants for brain protection.

### Vitamin E

Vitamin E is your body's most active antioxidant in the fatty (lipid) parts of your cells, which is why it is so important in the brain. It protects fatty cell membranes, neutralizes free radicals, and interrupts the oxidative process. Taking vitamin E supplements will help protect your cells against the destructive onslaught of free radicals and just may avert memory problems.

In the *Journal of the American Geriatrics Society,* Austrian researchers reported on a study of 1,769 people from the ages of fifty to seventy-five. They found that individuals with low blood levels of vitamin E performed more poorly on tests of cognitive function than those with high levels of the vitamin. The top-scoring individuals also had higher levels of beta-carotene, another antioxidant, but the difference in their levels and those of the low scorers was not statistically significant.

In animal studies, vitamin E has been shown to reduce the degeneration of cells in the hippocampus (the area of the brain that routes short-term memories to long-term storage) after injury to that area. In test-tube studies, vitamin E reduces neuron death associated with beta amyloid, the protein that causes senile plaques in the brains of patients with Alzheimer's disease. And supplements of this vitamin have been explored as a therapy for slowing the progression of Alzheimer's disease.

In a 1997 study published in the *New England Journal of Medicine,* 341 patients with Alzheimer's disease were treated for two years with either 2,000 milligrams of vitamin E, 10 milligrams of selegiline (a drug primarily used to treat Parkinson's disease), both vitamin E and selegiline, or a placebo. Researchers found that vitamin E alone slowed the progression of the disease more than selegiline alone or a combination of the two. This treatment kept several of the patients out of nursing homes and delayed expected milestones in the disease for up to seven months. One of the researchers, Dr. Carl Cotman, head of the Institute of Brain Aging and Dementia at the University of California, Irvine, stated in an interview, "This [vitamin E] is the first thing that really seems to put the brakes on Alzheimer's. And it's inexpensive, easily available, and safe, for the most part."

SUGGESTED DOSAGE: *A minimum of 800 international units of vitamin E daily. For those with Alzheimer's disease, the recommended dose is 2,000 international units. This is the amount that was used in the study above. Look for a supplement with natural d-alpha tocopherol (or d-alpha tocopheryl), preferably with mixed beta, delta, and gamma tocopherols. Avoid synthetic vitamin E, which is labeled as dl-alpha tocopherol (or dl-alpha tocopheryl).*

## Vitamin C

While vitamin E is the pre-eminent antioxidant of the fatty portions of the cells, vitamin C is the top gun in the watery areas. Vitamin C is obviously important to the brain and central nervous system because its concentration in the brain is fifteen times higher than elsewhere in the body. In addition to its antioxidant activity, vitamin C is involved in the production of several neurotransmitters, including acetylcholine, dopamine, and norepinephrine.

Numerous studies have demonstrated that this important nutrient is a predictable indicator of mental status in people of all ages. In one study, students were grouped by vitamin C blood levels, and their IQs were measured on standard tests. The IQs of the students with high vitamin C levels averaged five points greater than those of students with low levels. Both groups were given vitamin C supplements daily for six months. When they were retested, the students who had initially had low vitamin C status had a mean increase in IQ of 3.54 points, while the other group's IQs remained the same. The use of supplemental vitamin C to treat memory disorders is now being explored.

SUGGESTED DOSAGE: *Begin with 500 milligrams of vitamin C daily, gradually building the dosage to 2,500 milligrams over a two- to three-week period. Some may consider this to be a mega-dose, but my reasoning for this amount is simple. Somewhere along the evolutionary road, humans and other primates lost their ability to produce vitamin C. Almost all other species make their own supplies of this vital nutrient. According to calculations by Dr. Linus Pauling, they do so in amounts that, pound for pound, would equal 2,300 to 9,000 milligrams a day for a human. Given that you'll get some vitamin C in your diet, I feel that 2,500 milligrams is a reasonable supplemental dose. I suggest building up to that level gradually, as vitamin C causes gastrointestinal distress in some people.*

## Vitamin A and Beta-Carotene

Like vitamin E, vitamin A is a fat-soluble antioxidant that plays an important role in the brain. Beta-carotene, a carotenoid, is a precursor of vitamin A and is converted in the body into vitamin A as needed. The developing brain of the fetus depends on adequate amounts of vitamin A, and new research suggests that this nutrient is involved in brain function throughout life. Vitamin A has been described by Dr. Ronald Evans of the Salk Institute for Biological Studies in La Jolla, California, as "a type of molecular key that unlocks one of the most powerful functions of the human brain," learning. Dr. Evans and others are particularly concerned about the estimated 190 million children around the world who have vitamin A deficiencies.

SUGGESTED DOSAGE: *5,000 international units of vitamin A daily. (Because vitamin A is fat-soluble and can build up in the tissues, do not take over 10,000 international units without consulting your physician.) Also, add 15,000 international units of beta-carotene to your supplement program.*

## Coenzyme $Q_{10}$

Slow, sluggish, lethargic, dull—this is how you feel when you're tired and your energy level is low. This same state could describe what happens at the cellular level when your mitochondria, the powerhouses that fuel each of your cells, do not produce adequate energy. The result is a general slowdown in the cells and decrease in optimal function. One nutrient that is essential for energy production in every cell of your body is coenzyme $Q_{10}$ ($CoQ_{10}$). Like a spark plug, it jump-starts this energy transfer in the mitochondria. Without adequate supplies of $CoQ_{10}$, the energy output slows down. This is particularly detrimental for the brain, which is an energy guzzler and depends on a ready source of fuel.

In addition to improving energy production, coenzyme $Q_{10}$ has other beneficial effects in the brain. It has potent antioxidant activity and appears to protect the mitochondria against neurotoxins. It is being studied as a therapy for both Huntington's disease, an inherited disorder characterized by chronic degeneration and death of neurons, and Parkinson's disease, another neurodegenerative condition. One small study published in *The Lancet* showed that $CoQ_{10}$, in combination with vitamin $B_6$ and iron, actually delayed the progression of Alzheimer's disease by one and a half to two years.

Although it is neither a vitamin nor a mineral, coenzyme $Q_{10}$ is worthy of addition into a preventive nutritional supplementation program.

SUGGESTED DOSAGE: *A minimum dose of 60 milligrams of $CoQ_{10}$ daily (although four or five times this amount is common). $CoQ_{10}$ is better absorbed when taken with a little fat-containing food. Sold as an individual supplement, $CoQ_{10}$ is not a part of most multivitamin and mineral preparations.*

## Memory-Enhancing Minerals

Minerals are vital for our health and well-being. The seven major minerals are calcium, chloride, magnesium, phosphorus, potassium, sodium, and sulfur. The eleven minerals considered minor or trace (they are required in minute amounts) are boron, chromium, copper, iodine, iron, manganese, molybdenum, selenium, silicon, vanadium, and zinc. Although all of these minerals are necessary for optimal health, and it is important to take a daily supplement that contains the bulk of them, two in particular—magnesium and zinc—are especially important for their roles in brain function.

### Magnesium

Magnesium is a powerhouse of a mineral. It is involved in energy production, growth, sleep, wound healing, and muscle function. Magnesium is essential for normal functioning of the heart and cardiovascular system. It normalizes heartbeat and relaxes the muscular walls of the blood vessels, thus improving blood flow and lowering blood pressure. I strongly recommend magnesium for all my patients with heart disease. Because of its normalizing actions on the circulatory system, magnesium is beneficial to the brain. Without adequate blood flow to the brain, you've got big problems. Glucose, oxygen, and other nutrients are delivered via the blood, so good circulation is key to optimal cognitive function.

Magnesium has other more specific roles in the brain. When levels of this mineral are extremely low, which sometimes happens with patients taking diuretics, it may result in confusion, delirium, seizures, and even coma. There has even been specula-

TABLE 4.1. VITAMIN AND MINERAL RECOMMENDATIONS
FOR OPTIMAL BRAIN FUNCTION

| Vitamin/Mineral | Suggested Daily Dosage |
|---|---|
| Vitamin A | 5,000 international units |
| Beta-carotene | 15,000 international units |
| Vitamin $B_1$ (thiamin) | 50 milligrams |
| Vitamin $B_3$ (niacin) | 100 milligrams |
| Vitamin $B_5$ (pantothenic acid) | 50 milligrams |
| Vitamin $B_6$ (pyridoxine) | 75 milligrams |
| Vitamin $B_{12}$ | 100 micrograms |
| Vitamin C | 2,500 milligrams |
| Vitamin E | 800 international units |
| Choline | 425 milligrams* |
| Folic acid | 400 micrograms |
| Magnesium | 500 milligrams |
| Zinc | 30 milligrams |

* The recommended choline dosage for pregnant women is 450 milligrams; for nursing mothers, the recommended dosage is 550 milligrams.

tion that very low brain levels of magnesium are involved in Alzheimer's disease. As seen in Chapter 3, deposits of aluminum are found in the neurons of patients with this disease. We now know that these same neurons have very low concentrations of magnesium. One theory is that it isn't the aluminum itself that causes dementia, but rather its effects on blocking the actions of magnesium in the brain.

Magnesium deficiencies are common in this country, especially among older people.

SUGGESTED DOSAGE: *500 milligrams of magnesium daily, balanced with 1,000 milligrams of calcium. (In order to be effective, calcium and magnesium must be taken in a 2:1 or 1:1 ratio.)*

## Zinc

Important for the brain, zinc is a trace mineral that also has positive effects on the cardiovascular system. Zinc stabilizes cellular membranes, especially in the blood vessels, and is required for proper functioning of the immune system. It is also involved in smell, taste, and vision. Zinc deficiencies have been associated with memory loss and disorientation in elderly people. It may also be a factor in Alzheimer's disease, as levels of this important mineral are depleted in patients with this disease.

Several studies have shown that supplementing with zinc improves memory and recall in older patients with cognitive problems. In one study, ten patients with Alzheimer's disease were given 27 milligrams of zinc daily. Eight of the ten showed improved memory, communication, and understanding, and the improvements of one seventy-nine-year-old were described as "unbelievable."

**SUGGESTED DOSAGE:** *30 milligrams of zinc daily.*

## SUMMING IT UP

Although I've described the best studied of the vitamins and minerals that protect your brain, others are likely involved. My advice to you is to take a high-dose, broad-based multivitamin and mineral supplement to make sure you get adequate amounts of these and other nutrients involved in brain function and overall health maintenance.

STEP 3

# Restore Memory
# With Herbs

*S usie is a very successful hairstylist. Her success is due to her profes-
sional skills—she's a great hairdresser with thirty years experience—as well as her people skills. She treats all of her clients like old
friends. She always remembers the details of their lives, asks about their
family members by name, and never has to be reminded about their likes
and dislikes. Remarkably, she's always been able to store these details in
her head. While the other stylists in her shop keep notes on their clients
and services, Susie just remembers them.*

*About the time Susie turned forty-nine, she began to notice memo-
ry lapses. Small details, such as a child's name or where the client had
gone on vacation, would sometimes escape her. These were not serious
lapses, and in all likelihood no one noticed them but her. But to Susie,
they were bothersome. She started taking Ginkgo biloba, which she had
heard about from one of her clients. She thought she felt a little sharper
but didn't notice anything dramatic until six months later, when she
ran out of the herb. All of a sudden, the memory problems returned and
she began forgetting little things again. She is back on ginkgo and is
thoroughly convinced that it has improved her memory and made her
feel sharper and quicker.*

I've been recommending herbs at my medical clinic for over
twenty years, and I've witnessed firsthand their potential in
maintaining and restoring health. I've followed the growing body
of scientific research that confirms the effectiveness of herbal
remedies and identifies some of their key compounds. Based on
this research, we know what traditional societies have known for
millennia—herbs work. But now we also know how they work.

In this chapter you'll learn about *Ginkgo biloba*—a remarkable
herb that has the ability to sharpen your memory, help you focus

and concentrate better, and improve your mental edge. Other herbs that improve mental energy and overall cognitive function are presented as well. But first, it's important to learn a few general guidelines in choosing and selecting herbs. If you're like most people, you're probably not sure which herbs to take, or when and how to take them. You might be worried about possible side effects and other safety issues, and you may not know how to select a quality product. I sympathize. There's a lot of contradictory information out there. An herb may be positioned by one "authority" as a cure-all, and dismissed by another "expert" as ineffective and dangerous. Solid, trustworthy advice is hard to come by.

## HOW TO SELECT AND USE HERBS

We are in the midst of an herbal renaissance as Americans rediscover the age-old therapeutic powers of herbs. Sales of herbs are skyrocketing. They're sold everywhere from health food stores and pharmacies to discount stores and airport gift shops. Manufacturers of herbs and other nutritional supplements are forbidden by law to state on their products what they should be used for and how they will benefit health. This leaves consumers in the dark. Here are a few guidelines to assist you in your selection and use of herbs.

### Choose Cultivated, Organic Herbs

Harvesting herbs from their natural environment is called wild crafting. You might think herbs collected in this way would be preferable to cultivated herbs—those grown by commercial farming methods. But wild crafting has led to the near-extinction of certain herbs and the degradation of fragile ecosystems like the rainforests. Most of the herbal supplements you find in stores are cultivated varieties. They have fewer environmental and genetic variations because growing conditions can be better controlled. As a result, there is more consistency in the final product. I recommend you choose herbs that have been grown organically and screened for harmful pesticides. If you do use wild-crafted herbs, make sure that they are not endangered species.

## Use the Best Herbal Forms

You'll find that herbs come in several forms. *Bulk herbs* are herbs used as they occur in nature, such as peppermint leaves, chamomile flowers, garlic cloves, and ginger root. Bulk herbs can be ground into powders and formed into tablets or put into capsules. Or they can be steeped in boiling water and made into teas called *infusions*. Although bulk herbs, infusions, and powdered herbs offer some benefits, they vary significantly in quality and strength. They are, therefore, not a very reliable way to get a predictable and effective dose of the active ingredients in the herb.

*Extracts* are concentrated forms of whole herbs, and they come in three forms—tinctures, liquid extracts, and solid extracts. *Tinctures* are prepared by soaking the herb in a solvent such as water or alcohol, then pressing out the solution. A tincture's strength is measured in terms of its concentration. A typical tincture is a 1:5 concentration—it contains five times as much solvent as herbal material. Because they contain so much solvent in comparison to the amount of herb, tinctures are the weakest and least economical forms of herbal supplement. *Fluid extracts* are made by evaporating most of the solvent to yield a 1:1 concentration of herb to solvent. A typical liquid extract is five times as strong as a tincture made from the same solution. In *solid extracts,* the solvent is completely removed, making this extract even more concentrated than the fluid variety. The strength of a solid extract is measured in terms of grams of crude herb per grams of extract. For example, in a 5:1 concentration, five grams of the herb are used to produce one gram of the extract. So 200 milligrams of a solid extract contains the equivalent of 1,000 milligrams of a bulk herb.

I recommend that you choose solid herbal extracts whenever possible. They are the most concentrated form, and they have the greatest chemical stability. In addition, they are the most economical.

## Choose Extracts Standardized for Active Ingredients

One of the most important contributions scientific research has made to consumers and the herbal industry is the standardization of herbal extracts. Researchers have identified the active ingredients, or constituents, in each herb that give it its therapeutic powers. Scientific studies have also determined an effective dose of that active ingredient in herbal extracts. Manufacturers, therefore, are better able to evaluate the bulk herbs they purchase and adjust their concentrations to ensure that the finished products contain enough of the active constituents to be effective. These constituents are not isolated and sold as individual items—this would be contrary to the whole philosophy of herbal medicine. There are likely other important ingredients in the herb not yet identified as being active constituents. Furthermore, there is a synergy in nature. Things often work better together than on their own. Standardized herbal extracts contain everything nature put in them, including a specified amount of the most important constituents.

This has made it possible for manufacturers to guarantee the potency of their products. It also gives you, the consumer, the confidence of knowing that you are getting what you pay for. Before the advent of standardization, shopping for herbs was a guessing game. (I've read several studies in which herbal supplements were analyzed and found to contain little or none of the herb identified on the label!) For example, let's say you are shopping for the herb feverfew, which is used for the prevention of migraine headaches. You go into a store and find, say, six different brands of feverfew. Some may be tablets, some may be capsules, and the potency of each may vary, but all of the products appear to be pretty much the same. How do you know which brand to choose? You may decide, all things appearing equal, to purchase the least expensive. Or you may be of the "you get what you pay for" school of thought and select the most expensive brand. Perhaps you're an old hand at herbs, and you have a favorite brand that you know is effective. Great, but you're in the minority. With so little information on the labels, there is nothing to guide you in your selection. Here's where standardization comes in.

We know that a phytochemical in feverfew called *parthenolide* gives the herb its headache-prevention properties. We also know from the research on feverfew that the most effective feverfew preparations contain 0.4- to 0.7-percent parthenolide. Therefore, a feverfew product standardized to contain 0.4- to 0.7-percent parthenolide is the most reliable product. Look for standardized extracts in all herbs. They're becoming more and more commonplace.

### Insist on Quality Control

Herbs should be thoroughly tested and analyzed during harvesting and manufacturing. When you're not sure about a product, don't be shy about calling the manufacturer and asking about quality control. At a minimum, the following three types of analysis should be done:

1. *Herbs should be chemically tested for identity.* Even experts can have difficulty identifying herbs within the same family. Chemical testing is the only way to ensure that the herb is what it is represented to be.

2. *Herbs should be tested for potency.* Climactic conditions, soil quality, rainfall, and growing time all contribute to the potency of the harvested herb. Uniform potency from batch to batch must be ensured. If the herb is a standardized extract, sophisticated analytical techniques must be used to verify the level of active compounds in every bottle.

3. *All herbs should be screened for impurities and contaminants.* Even organic herbs should be tested for pesticides, heavy metals, and microbes.

Keep these points in mind when selecting your herbal supplement. You owe it to yourself to get what you pay for—quality products.

---

## Use Herbs Properly

Herbs are not like vitamins and minerals, which I recommend for people of all ages to take for overall health. Herbs should be viewed as targeted therapies used to prevent or treat specific conditions. Furthermore, unlike vitamins and minerals, all herbal preparations are not taken in the same manner. Some are appropriate for daily use, while others require periodic breaks. A few herbs interact with prescription drugs, and some are not advisable if you have certain health problems. Before taking any herbal treatments, do your homework. Make sure you take herbs as recommended, carefully considering possible allergic reactions and interactions with drugs you may be taking. Never exceed the recommended doses. Pregnant or nursing women should approach all herbs with caution. And all herbs should be kept out of reach of children.

## NATURE'S MEMORY BOOSTERS

Some of the most exciting recent medical findings involve the power of herbs. Garlic, for instance, has been shown to lower cholesterol and blood pressure. Horse chestnut has been used to help eliminate varicose veins. Black cohosh is effective in easing some of the discomforts of menopause. St. John's wort elevates mood. And some herbs, such as *Ginkgo biloba,* ginseng, Huperzine A, and vinpocetine, have been clinically proven to preserve and restore memory. Let's take a closer look at these herbal brain boosters.

## Ginkgo biloba

If I could recommend only one herbal supplement for optimizing brain function, it would be *Ginkgo biloba.* The ginkgo tree, dating back over 200 million years, is one of the oldest living plant species on the planet. Extremely hardy, ginkgo trees are resistant to insects, pollution, and disease. Their leaves have been used for various medicinal purposes for centuries. A 5,000-year-old Chinese medical text describes ginkgo as "benefiting the brain."

Today, ginkgo is commonly used in Europe, where physicians write prescriptions for herbs and insurance companies pay for them. In fact, over 10 million prescriptions are written throughout the world for ginkgo each year for the treatment of circulatory disorders, depression, memory loss, and other signs of cognitive decline.

Extracts from the leaves of this tree contain phytochemicals called *ginkgo flavone glycosides* and *terpene lactones*, which give ginkgo its remarkable medicinal value. These phytochemicals have powerful antioxidant activity, as well as stabilizing effects on cellular membranes. Their activities are particularly visible in the brain. As discussed earlier, 60 percent of your brain is fat, and ginkgo assists vitamin E and other antioxidants in protecting these fatty tissues from free-radical damage. Ginkgo also enhances the production of neurotransmitters and normalizes acetylcholine receptors. Furthermore, this herb enhances the utilization of glucose, providing additional energy for the brain.

As remarkable as these benefits may seem, ginkgo's greatest attribute is its ability to improve blood flow to the smallest of capillaries. It is, therefore, useful as a treatment for problems that result from impaired circulation, such as erectile dysfunction in men, vascular problems in the legs, and memory and cognitive declines. *Ginkgo biloba* mildly dilates blood vessel walls and inhibits the actions of a substance called platelet activating factor (PAF), which causes platelets to clump together. The overall result is improved circulation, and nowhere is this as important as in the brain, which requires a constant supply of glucose and oxygen.

Of all the cells in your body, brain cells are the most apt to suffer the consequences of oxygen deprivation. Many symptoms of reduced blood flow to the brain—a condition known as *cerebral vascular insufficiency*—are precisely those of age-related cognitive impairment and more serious dementia. These symptoms may include memory and concentration difficulties, absentmindedness, confusion, lack of energy, depression, anxiety, dizziness, tinnitus (ringing in the ears), and headache. Supplementing with *Ginkgo biloba* may prevent and even reverse these symptoms by improving blood flow and ensuring adequate delivery of nutrients and oxygen to the brain.

Several clinical trials have examined ginkgo's effectiveness in the treatment of cerebral vascular insufficiency. In 1992, Europe's premier medical journal, *The Lancet*, published a review of ten well-controlled ginkgo trials. Researchers Jos Kleijnin and Paul Knipschild, of the University of Limburg in the Netherlands, found through these studies that taking *Ginkgo biloba* extracts resulted in significant improvements in memory, concentration, energy, and mood. Test subjects taking ginkgo also reported less confusion and dizziness, and fewer headaches. This analysis further described how the electrical brain activity of elderly patients in two of the trials, as measured by electroencephalograms (EEGs), returned to normal with ginkgo supplementation.

A more recent French study enrolled eighteen subjects between age sixty and eighty, who had slight cognitive impairment. In this double-blind, placebo-controlled study, patients were administered one of three protocols—320 milligrams ginkgo, 600 milligrams ginkgo, or a placebo. One hour later, the subjects took a battery of tests to determine their speed of information processing. The results were astounding. After treatment with ginkgo, the patients' scores improved so dramatically that they were close to the scores of healthy young people. When the groups were crossed over—the people who initially took the placebo were given ginkgo and vice versa—those taking ginkgo again scored much better. This study indicates that ginkgo may significantly benefit memory, even in people who have already demonstrated some memory loss. Interestingly, there were no significant differences between the two groups taking different amounts of ginkgo. Performance improved similarly in both groups.

Several studies suggest that ginkgo extract may even be effective for patients with Alzheimer's disease. The *Journal of the American Medical Association* published a study in the October 1997 issue showing that ginkgo slows cognitive decline and improves attention span and memory in Alzheimer's patients when taken over a three-month period. Other studies, which were analyzed in the November 1998 issue of *Archives of Neurology,* have reached the same conclusion. The studies reviewed in this analysis involved a total of 424 patients with Alzheimer's disease who were administered tests of cognitive function, then given either 120 to 240 milligrams of ginkgo or a placebo daily for three to six months. When they were retested, the patients taking ginkgo experienced a 3-percent improvement in their scores on memory and learning tests, compared to the patients taking a placebo.

*Ginkgo biloba* also improves memory and sharpens cognitive function in young, healthy people. For best results, I recommend taking ginkgo every day. Look for a standardized extract containing 24-percent ginkgo flavone glycosides and 6-percent terpene lactones. Some products are also standardized for a minimum of 0.8-percent ginkgolide B. The recommended dosage is 60 milligrams twice a day with meals.

As with many herbal agents, ginkgo's effects will not be apparent overnight. It may take up to twelve weeks before you notice benefits. This herb is extremely safe, and although side effects are rare, it may cause mild gastrointestinal upset, headache, or allergic skin reactions in sensitive individuals. If you are taking an MAO inhibitor or a blood thinner like warfarin (Coumadin), please consult your physician before taking ginkgo. Also, check with your doctor if you are pregnant or nursing before using this herb. *Ginkgo biloba* is not recommended for children.

## Ginseng

Ginseng is another herbal extract that benefits the brain. It helps improve memory and concentration by combating the negative effects of stress on your brain. Ginseng has been shown to improve performance on a variety of tasks that require concentration and focus, especially under conditions of stress.

In one study, telegraph operators taking ginseng demonstrated improved concentration and made few mistakes. In another study, students were able to sharpen their focus and score better on tests. Ginseng is presented in greater detail in Step 7 in the discussion on improving memory through effective stress management.

## Vinpocetine

Vinpocetine, from the lesser periwinkle plant (*Vinca minor*), has remarkable restorative powers on brain function. It improves energy production in neurons and blood flow to the brain. Clinical studies have shown it to be an effective therapy in cerebral vascular insufficiency. It also improves memory in young, healthy study subjects. More information on vinpocetine is given in Step 10 on "smart" nutrients.

## Huperzine A

Huperzine A is an extract from club moss (*Huperzia serrata*). It elevates levels of the neurotransmitter acetylcholine by blocking the enzyme that breaks it down. This nutrient appears to be equally as effective as, if not more effective than, the prescription drugs marketed for the treatment of Alzheimer's disease. Considered a "smart" nutrient, Huperzine A is discussed in greater detail in Step 10.

## SUMMING IT UP

Don't wait for your doctor to recommend *Ginkgo biloba* or the other brain-boosting herbs presented in Step 3. Although these herbs are safe, effective therapies for enhancing memory in healthy individuals and improving cognitive function in those with memory loss, the medical establishment tends to ignore them. Please do not mistake their indifference for an herb's lack of efficacy or scientific backing. It is simply a typical response in the conventional medicine arena.

Now it's on to Step 4 of the program. There we will discuss the fats that nurture the brain.

Step 4

# Nurture Your Brain
# With Fats

*L*orenzo Odone was a bright, engaging little boy, the beloved son of an
Italian-American couple. The Odones' lives were turned upside
down in 1984, when Lorenzo, at the age of five, began to experience
behavior and memory problems. Over the next few months, his symptoms grew progressively more serious. He developed muscular weakness
and difficulties with speech, vision, and hearing, and eventually he was
bedridden and completely unable to speak.

Lorenzo was diagnosed with adrenoleukodystrophy (ALD), a rare
and often fatal disease of the brain. ALD is characterized by degeneration of the adrenal glands and the fatty myelin sheaths surrounding the
brain's nerve cells.

Refusing to accept their son's dire prognosis, Lorenzo's parents—
without much support from the medical establishment—embarked on a
frantic, focused search for a cure for their son's "incurable" condition.
What they discovered, and research has since borne out, is that ALD is
caused by a genetic defect that impairs the body's ability to break down
certain fats. These fats accumulate in the brain and adrenal glands, and
they destroy normal tissues.

By feeding Lorenzo certain types of fats, the Odones discovered that
his condition was able to be halted (but, unfortunately, not reversed).
Lorenzo is alive today, and able to communicate through the use of ges-
tures. "Lorenzo's oil," however, has prevented the progression of ALD
in Lorenzo and countless other children. A foundation established by the
Odones is devoted to researching this condition further.

Fat has a terrible reputation. It's synonymous with cellulite,
potbellies, and love handles. It is blamed for heart disease, cancer, and other ills. Americans are constantly advised by health
experts to eat less fat, which has spawned an entire industry of

low-fat and fat-free foods. While it's true that too much of the wrong kinds of fat, particularly saturated fats and the trans fatty acids discussed in Step 1, can have serious health consequences, your brain absolutely requires certain fats for optimal function (as Lorenzo's story illustrates).

Before jumping into this chapter, I want to give you a heads up. You might find the material on the next few pages difficult to grasp. Don't worry. It doesn't mean that you're losing your mental edge. The subject of fats is very complicated, and it's hard to present without resorting to technical terminology. I have used abbreviations as much as possible to cut down on the scientific terminology (see inset on page 118), and I've done my best to keep it as short and simple as possible. On the other hand, why and how the fats you put into your mouth have such a profound influence on your brain is such an important, cutting-edge, and, in my opinion, fascinating subject that I want to explain it for those of you who want to scratch below the surface. We waded into the subject of fats in Step 1. Now, let's dive in!

## FAT AND HEALTH

Fats and oils, more technically called *lipids,* encompass a broad range of substances that share a common basic chemical structure. They are chains of carbon and hydrogen with one or more oxygen molecules, and their building blocks are called *fatty acids* (see inset on page 120). Let's briefly review the three major categories of fatty acids we get from the foods we eat—saturated, monounsaturated, and polyunsaturated fats.

*Saturated fatty acids* are found in meat, dairy products, and tropical oils. Because of their relatively stable chemical structure, saturated fatty acids are not very active biochemically. In other words, they cannot perform some of the important chemical functions in your body that other fatty acids can. While this type of fat is a structural component of all cell membranes, including brain cells, it is best to limit your intake of saturated fat. Your body is able to manufacture all you need. Too much saturated fat causes platelets in the blood to become sticky, impairing circulation and increasing the risk of heart attack. Saturated fatty acids may also be deposited inside artery walls and within organs, contributing to obesity, heart disease, and other degenerative conditions.

*Monounsaturated fatty acids,* which are abundant in olive, canola, almond, and peanut oil, have a less stable structure and are chemically more active than saturated fatty acids. These fats are also incorporated into the membranes of your cells, and they help keep your arteries supple and elastic. Like saturated fats, your body can produce monounsaturated fatty acids, so dietary sources are not critical. They are fine in moderation.

*Polyunsaturated fatty acids* are the most important fats for health because their chemical structure makes them the most biochemically active fats of all. Two polyunsaturated fatty acids that are particularly noteworthy are *linoleic acid (LA)* and *alpha-linolenic acid (ALA).* LA and ALA are called *essential fatty acids (EFAs)* because, unlike the other fats we've discussed thus far, they cannot be synthesized in the body. Furthermore, all of the other fats your body needs can be made from these EFAs.

The roles of EFAs are diverse. They are involved in energy production and the cellular transport of oxygen. They are an integral component of cell membranes—cell membranes formed in the absence of adequate EFAs lack the structural integrity of healthy cells. They are also required for proper growth and functioning of the brain, skin and hair, reproductive organs, liver and kidneys, and immune and cardiovascular systems. In addition, EFAs are precursors to prostaglandins, powerful hormone-like chemical messengers that regulate blood flow, the immune response, and inflammation.

We discussed the importance of balance between the two classes of EFAs in Step 1. Let me explain why this balance is so important for overall health. LA is an omega-6 fatty acid and a precursor to highly inflammatory prostaglandins that activate the immune system and cause swelling, increased sensitivity to pain, and thickening and clotting of the blood. ALA, an omega-3 fatty acid, is a precursor to another class of prostaglandins that have mild anti-inflammatory effects. The importance of maintaining a balance between these prostaglandins is obvious.

Omega-6 fatty acids are abundant in meats, dairy products,

## Cholesterol and Your Brain

Believe it or not, cholesterol—a dreaded word to most people—is a vital part of your brain. Cholesterol is a crucial component of all cell membranes, as it regulates their fluidity. For cell membranes to function at their best, they must be neither too stiff nor too soft. To maintain their ideal consistency, cholesterol is added to excessively fluid membranes or removed from overly stiff ones. One-fourth of the fat content of the myelin sheaths that protect and insulate axons is made up of cholesterol. Cholesterol is also the precursor of the steroid hormones, DHEA, pregnenolone, estrogen, progesterone, and testosterone, which affect brain function.

Important as cholesterol is, don't get the idea that it's beneficial to start eating steaks and cheese just to raise your cholesterol levels. Your body produces plenty of cholesterol on its own.

and vegetable oils that we commonly consume. The only dietary sources of the omega-3 fatty acids, however, are cold-water fish and flaxseed oil. And once you understand that inflammatory prostaglandins are also formed by fatty acids present in meat and dairy products, you can imagine how common imbalances are. We need to bring this back into balance, and that's why I've devoted this rung of my 10-step program to boosting levels of the omega-3 fatty acids in your brain.

## FATTY ACIDS AND YOUR BRAIN

Almost one-third of the fat in your brain is polyunsaturated. The two most abundant of these brain fats are *docosahexaenoic acid (DHA)* and *arachidonic acid (AA)*. AA is an omega-6 fatty acid, formed from the essential fatty acid LA. Because it is also found in meat and dairy products, most of us get plenty, if not too much AA. And while AA is an important fatty acid in your brain, when it is out of balance with the omega-3 fatty acids, it has a dark side—it stimulates excess production of inflammatory prostaglandins, as described above.

DHA is an omega-3 fatty acid, one of two important fatty

acids derived from the essential fatty acid ALA. (DHA should not be confused with the hormone DHEA, which we will discuss in Step 9.) The other is *eicosapentaenoic acid (EPA),* which benefits the brain primarily by improving blood flow and the delivery of oxygen and nutrients. However, there is little EPA in the brain. The brain's most important omega-3 fatty acid is DHA.

## DHA: The Smart Fat

DHA is a long-chain polyunsaturated fatty acid with six double bonds, making it a hotbed of electric and chemical activity. DHA is concentrated in the synaptic gaps between axons and dendrites, where communication between nerve cells takes place. It is also abundant in the neurons' mitochondria, as well as the light receptors in the eyes. The cerebral cortex, "the crowning achievement of evolution" where reasoning, learning, and memory abide, is loaded with DHA.

When your brain doesn't have enough DHA, it substitutes other fatty acids in its place. Even trans fatty acids, the chemically corrupted, harmful fats discussed in Step 1, have been discovered in brain cell membranes in the places that are usually filled with DHA. When brain cells are forced to settle for these inferior fatty acids, they are unable to function at their best.

DHA plays a particularly crucial role in the brain development of infants and children. Together with other long-chain polyunsaturated fatty acids, DHA accumulates in the fetal brain late in pregnancy, and continues to accumulate during an infant's first few months of life. Human breast milk contains much more of these critical fats than cow's milk or formula, so babies who are not breastfed have lower levels of these important nutrients. Researchers have determined that these important fatty acids affect intelligence in infancy and perhaps later in life.

In a 1998 study published in *The Lancet,* Scottish researchers placed forty-four healthy babies into two groups. The formula of one group was supplemented with long-chain polyunsaturated fatty acids for the first four months of their lives. The other group was fed regular formula. At the age of ten months, the babies were given tests of problem solving, such as finding a hidden toy.

# Abbreviations

The following abbreviations are used throughout this chapter to minimize the technical terminology.

**AA    Arachidonic acid.** The most abundant omega-6 fatty acid in the brain; excessive amounts may be converted into harmful inflammatory prostaglandins. Abundant in meat and dairy products.

**ALA    Alpha-linolenic acid.** An omega-3 essential fatty acid and a precursor to DHA and EPA. Found in flaxseed oil.

**DHA    Docosahexaenoic acid.** The most important omega-3 fatty acid in the brain. It is vital for optimal brain function. Best dietary source is cold-water fish.

**EFA    Essential fatty acid.** Important fatty acids that the body is unable to manufacture itself. EFAs must come from dietary sources or supplements.

**EPA    Eicosapentaenoic acid.** An omega-3 fatty acid that enhances circulation. Found in cold-water fish.

**LA    Linoleic acid.** An omega-6 essential fatty acid and precursor to AA. Abundant in safflower, sunflower, soybean, walnut, and sesame oil.

**PC    Phosphatidyl choline.** A constituent of nerve cell membranes and a source of choline. It is necesssary for the production of acetylcholine. Found in lecithin, eggs, and soy products.

**PS    Phosphatidyl serine.** A component of nerve cell membranes. Best taken in supplement form.

The babies whose formulas had been supplemented with the fatty acids displayed significantly superior problem-solving abilities in locating the hidden toy. Their memories and attention spans were also better than those of the babies who had been fed regular formula. The researchers concluded that supplementation with these EFAs was important for the development of early intelligence.

DHA remains the most important brain fat throughout life. Low levels of DHA are associated with an increased risk of memory loss. Dr. Michael A. Schmidt reports in *Smart Fats* that, according to data collected in the long-term Framingham Heart Study, adults with low levels of DHA have a greater likelihood of developing dementia in their later years. Other studies have indicated these adults are twice as likely to develop dementia as those with high levels of DHA. And a 1997 study demonstrated that low DHA blood levels are an important risk factor for Alzheimer's disease.

In Japan, where the benefits of DHA are widely recognized, many foods are nutritionally fortified with DHA. Students there reportedly take DHA pills prior to examinations to enhance their performance. Japanese studies have shown that supplemental DHA sharpens memory in patients with dementia and depression and improves behavior and speech in those with Alzheimer's disease.

How can you restore the proper balance between omega-6 and omega-3 fatty acids and ensure that you're feeding your brain the fats it needs for optimal functioning? Supplement with omega-3 oils and, more specifically, DHA. Fish oil capsules, the most common type of omega-3 supplements, contain DHA (each 1,000-milligram capsule has approximately 120 milligrams of DHA). ALA, the omega-3 essential fatty acid, is also abundant in flaxseed and flaxseed oil, but it must be converted in the body to DHA. This makes flax oil less effective in raising DHA levels than fish oils. Algae-derived DHA supplements are another option. (Fish get their DHA from eating algae.)

For the health of your brain, daily supplementation of DHA is recommended from one of the following sources:

❑ 100 to 200 milligrams of isolated DHA daily.

❑ 1,000-milligram capsule of fish oil, twice a day.

❑ $1/_4$ cup freshly ground flaxseed, or $1^1/_2$ to 3 tablespoons of flaxseed oil daily.

Because these fats are subject to free-radical damage, I suggest taking 800 international units of vitamin E per day. This will help

# What Exactly Is a Fatty Acid?

Fatty acids are the building blocks of fats. Double bonds (=) are what make them biochemically active. Double bonds produce a slight negative electric charge, attract oxygen, and increase inter-action with other substances. They also give the molecule a curved (cis) shape, which gives it fluidity. Saturated fats are filled or saturated with hydrogen atoms and, therefore, have only single bonds (–) between their carbon atoms (C). Saturated fatty acids are relatively stable and inert. Monounsaturated fatty acids con-tain one double bond (=), making them more biochemically active than saturated fats. Polyunsaturated fatty acids, which have more than one double bond, are the most biochemically active of all.

C–C–C–C–C–C–C–C–C–C–C–C–C–C–C–C–C–C
**Saturated Fatty Acid**
*Has only single bonds (–) between carbon atoms.*

C–C–C–C–C–C–C–C–C=C–C–C–C–C–C–C–C–C
**Monounsaturated Fatty Acid**
*Has one double bond (=) between carbon atoms.*

C–C–C–C–C–C=C–C–C=C–C–C–C–C–C–C–C–C
**Polyunsaturated Fatty Acid**
*Has more than one double bond (=) between carbon atoms.*

protect these fragile oils from oxidation (see Step 2 for more infor-mation on antioxidants). DHA supplementation is especially important for pregnant women, nursing mothers, strict vegetari-ans, and people over the age of forty-five.

## PHOSPHOLIPIDS

Phospholipids, also known as phosphatides, differ from other fats in that they contain a phosphate group, which is attached to the fatty acid—hence the name, phospholipid. Phospholipids form the membranes that surround every cell. They serve as the cell's structural support and create a barrier that protects it. Phospholipids also act as sentries, controlling what goes into and out of a cell. And they facilitate communication with other cells. Two important phospholipids in the brain are phosphatidyl serine and phosphatidyl choline.

## Phosphatidyl Serine

One of the most plentiful phospholipids in brain tissue is phosphatidyl serine (PS). In addition to being a major component of neuronal membranes, PS performs other important functions in the brain. It is involved in both the receiving and transmitting ends of neurons. (It increases the activity of the receptors on the dendrites and activates the release of neurotransmitters from the axons.) PS also stimulates the production of the neurotransmitters dopamine, serotonin, and norepinephrine.

Supplemental PS easily crosses the blood-brain barrier and is incorporated into brain cells. Almost 3,000 studies on PS exist in the medical literature. Hundreds of animal studies reveal that PS prevents age-related declines in memory and learning. More than sixty clinical studies involving humans have been published, nearly a third of which were well-controlled double-blind studies comparing PS to a placebo. These studies demonstrated that PS is a safe supplement that assists in normalizing brain biochemistry and improving brain function.

One 1991 study included 149 patients from age fifty to seventy who had been experiencing minor memory lapses, concentration difficulties, and other signs of age-related memory impairment. The patients were placed in two groups. One group was given 300 milligrams of PS every day for twelve weeks, and the other was given a placebo. Both groups took tests of cognitive function before beginning supplementation, and again every three weeks throughout the study. The results were astounding. Those who took PS showed improvement in several areas—recalling telephone numbers, learning and placing names with faces, memorizing paragraphs, finding misplaced objects, and concentrating while performing tasks, reading, and chatting. Perhaps most important, the study subjects who had the greatest memory deficits at the start of the study showed the most significant improvements. According to principal investigator, Dr. Thomas H. Crook, III, supplementing with PS took twelve years off these patients' ages, in terms of mental function. In other words, they performed as well on cognitive function tests as people twelve years younger!

In addition to this remarkable study, other clinical trials have shown that supplemental PS improves several components of cognitive function, including concentration, attention span, and memorization skills in individuals with minor memory impairment. Other studies have shown that patients with more serious memory problems, including Alzheimer's disease, benefit from this supplement, as well. And still other studies have indicated that the benefits of PS continue after the supplement has been discontinued.

Phosphatidyl serine comes from two sources, bovine and soy. Although most of the initial research was done with bovine PS, concerns about *bovine spongiform encephalopathy* (mad cow disease) have made soy-source PS the preferred choice. And according to Dr. Crook, not only is soy PS safer, it's equally effective.

The recommended starting dosage of PS is 200 to 300 milligrams daily, tapering down to 100 milligrams after one month.

## Phosphatidyl Choline, Choline, and Lecithin

Phosphatidyl serine is not the only phospholipid in the brain. Another important component of nerve cell membranes is phosphatidyl choline (PC)—facilitator of intercellular communication. These two phospholipids are similar in structure, but PS contains the amino acid serine, and PC contains choline. As explained in the discussion of the B-complex vitamins in Step 2, choline is critical for the developing brain of the fetus. Studies have demonstrated an intellectual boost in animals that received adequate amounts of choline in utero from their mothers' diets and after birth from breast milk.

Choline is also a building block of acetylcholine—one of the brain's most important neurotransmitters. By taking a B-complex or multivitamin that contains choline, you will be providing your brain with the raw materials to manufacture both acetylcholine and PC.

Phosphatidyl choline may also be directly supplemented for additional protection. It is abundant in lecithin, which is found in egg yolks and soybean oil. Whether it's from dietary sources, lecithin, or isolated supplements, phosphatidyl choline easily enters brain tissue, where it is used by cell membranes or converted into acetylcholine. Because PC doesn't cause the gastrointestinal distress that sometimes accompanies choline supplementation, it can be taken in higher doses. The recommended PC dose is 50 to 100 milligrams. These supplements should always be taken with vitamin $B_5$ (pantothenic acid), which is required in the synthesis of acetylcholine, and contained in most multivitamins.

Citicoline, one of the "smart" nutrients, also improves brain function by boosting choline and PC levels. Citicoline is discussed in Step 10.

## SUMMING IT UP

As you can see, the fats you ingest have a profound influence on your brain. Although you can get these important brain fats through diet, I strongly suggest taking them in supplement form to ensure that you are getting adequate levels.

So far, we have covered the dietary measures and nutritional supplements that are necessary for peak cognitive function. Next, we'll be moving on to another area in maintaining mental sharpness—exercise.

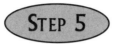

# Exercise for Peak Mental Performance

*B*ill *loved to play cards, especially blackjack, and he was good at it. Like a pro, he was able to "count cards"—remember all of the cards that come out during the game. As any gambler will tell you, counting cards is the only way to gain the edge consistently when playing blackjack. When Bill was in his early seventies, he moved into an assisted living facility, but he continued to play blackjack with the best of them. However, over time, he began having trouble counting and remembering cards. This bothered him so much that he just stopped playing. Since card playing had been Bill's main social outlet, he became reclusive and depressed.*

*While living at the facility, Bill had become more and more sedentary, and he began having trouble with his joints. He was enrolled in an exercise program with a physical therapist. For the first time in several years, he got outside on a regular basis, taking forty-five-minute walks with his therapist four days a week. He also engaged in supervised exercises in a gym. The regular exercise regimen switched on a light on in Bill's brain. His outlook improved dramatically, and he no longer felt depressed. He regained his former interests and renewed his social ties. At the end of his six-week exercise program, his memory had improved to the point that he was once again enjoying himself at cards, and cleaning up at the blackjack table.*

If we could bottle the benefits of physical exercise, we would have one of the most powerful remedies known to mankind. Regular, moderate exercise strengthens the heart, raises healthy HDL cholesterol levels, and decreases the risk of heart attack. It also improves circulation and lowers blood pressure. Exercise builds muscle, reduces fat, and helps normalize metabolism and weight. It strengthens the immune system, prevents migraine headaches, and reduces stress. Typically, those who exercise regularly live longer and have fewer heart attacks and a reduced incidence of some types of cancer. They have stronger bones, better developed muscles, and less body fat. Exercise is simply the healthiest habit you can acquire. You're no doubt aware of many of these benefits of exercise, but did you know that it is also good for your brain and mental functioning?

## SHARPEN YOUR MENTAL EDGE WITH EXERCISE

As discussed in earlier chapters, your brain is a ravenous consumer of glucose and oxygen. This small organ, which makes up about 2 percent of your total body weight, uses an incredible 25 percent of the oxygen you breathe. It is so dependent upon oxygen that if deprived of it for only a few minutes, brain cells die.

One way in which exercise benefits the brain is by increasing its access to oxygen and glucose. It does this in several ways. First, exercise strengthens the lungs and their capacity for oxygenating the blood. This ensures a constant supply of life-sustaining oxygen to the brain cells. Second, it makes the heart stronger and able to pump more oxygen- and nutrient-rich blood through the carotid arteries to your brain. Laboratory studies demonstrate that animals who are exercised vigorously develop more capillaries and have increased delivery of blood and nutrients around their neurons than sedentary animals. Third, exercise normalizes glucose metabolism, ensuring a steady stream of energy to the brain. As discussed in Step 1, if your brain doesn't have adequate glucose, your thinking will be impaired, and you'll feel tired, unfocused, and irritable.

According to Dharma Singh Khalsa, M.D., director of the Alzheimer's Prevention Foundation in Tucson and author of *Brain Longevity*, exercise also stimulates the production of an important substance called *nerve growth factor (NGF)*. As its name implies, NGF facilitates the growth of dendrites, the branchlike nerve endings that receive incoming signals and make intercellular communication possible. NGF also contributes to increased production of the neurotransmitters dopamine and acetylcholine, which are both critical for brain function and memory. In an experiment conducted at Johns Hopkins University, scientists gave older rats injections of NGF for three weeks, then ran them through mazes designed to test memory and learning. Their performance on these tests showed significant improvement, and new neurons sprouted up in the areas of the brain that received the NGF injections. At this time, NGF as a therapy for memory loss is still in the experimental stages. Exercise is not. Raise your own NGF levels by exercising regularly.

Another brain-boosting benefit of exercise is that it prompts the production of *endorphins*. Endorphins are natural chemicals that have an opiate-like effect in the body. In fact, the word endorphin comes from *endogenous*, which means "produced within," and *morphine*, a powerful painkiller and sedative. Endorphins are sometimes referred to as the "feel-good" neurotransmitters. Your body's production of endorphins begins after about twenty minutes of vigorous exercise and continues for hours thereafter. People who exercise regularly think more clearly, feel more alert and energetic, and have a markedly increased sense of well being. They also have better memories. I can personally attest to this. In 1995, I fulfilled a lifelong dream by riding a bicycle across the United States. It took ten weeks, and many of those 2,000-plus miles were grueling, but my memories of that trip are crystal clear. I can still smell the wildflowers growing on the side of the road, feel the early morning mist on my face and the wind on my back, and see the grandeur of the Cascade Mountains.

The positive effects of exercise on mental function have been borne out in several studies. Researchers at the Veterans' Medical Center in Salt Lake City, Utah, compared cognitive function of sedentary senior citizens to people of the same age who were put on an exercise program that included fifty minutes of brisk walking three times a week. After four months, participants were tested for reaction time, visual organization, memory, and mental flexibility. Not surprisingly, the exercisers scored higher than the sedentary group on reaction time. More interesting, however, was the fact that they also outperformed the nonexercisers on visual organization, memory, and mental flexibility.

Another study compared two groups of men. One group included fifty- to seventy-year-olds who played racquetball three times a week. The other group consisted of younger but inactive men. Guess who performed better on tests of mental acuity? Believe it or not, the older, more active men outperformed the young couch potatoes.

Exercise may even make you more creative. A 1997 study published in the *British Journal of Sports Medicine* tested sixty-three men and women who were divided into two groups. One group exercised, while the other group watched an uninspiring documentary film. The exercisers were further divided into two groups—one did very high-impact aerobics, and the other had a gentler exercise regimen. After the participants either exercised or watched the movie, they were asked to come up with unconventional ways to use a cardboard box or a tin can. Both the heavy and mild exercisers thought of more creative solutions to the problem than the sedentary group that had watched the movie. Mood in the exercisers also improved by 25 percent, although mood and creativity weren't necessarily linked.

## THE NUTS AND BOLTS OF EXERCISE

I could go on and on and give you the details of study after study, but they all have similar findings—exercise improves memory and sharpens mental edge. And we're not talking about running marathons or taking vigorous aerobics classes five days a week. Simply getting outside and walking or participating in any activity that gets you moving will do the trick. Whatever form of exercise you choose, do it for at least thirty minutes, three to five times a week—the ideal is forty-five minutes four days a week. Laying out a detailed exercise program is beyond the scope of this book, but I do want to give you the following guidelines for a safe and healthy exercise regimen.

### Get Ready, Get Set . . .

If you've been inactive, don't plunge wildly into a marathon-training program. Before you get started, especially if you are forty-five or older, get a thorough physical examination. This may seem like a costly, unnecessary step, but it is important. Your doctor is likely to make sure your heart responds normally to exercise. He or she may have you perform a stress test in which your heart is monitored while you exercise on a treadmill. This is a simple, noninvasive test, and if you haven't had one recently, it's time you did. Should any abnormalities be present, it's best to find out in the physician's office, rather than in the gym or on the track. If you have any joint problems or other physical concerns, discuss them with your doctor, who can make recommendations as to the best types of exercise for you.

Second, decide on what form of exercise you're going to do. Consider weather, facilities in your area, equipment you might need, your own physical condition, and above all, your personal preferences—if you don't enjoy it, the odds are you won't stick with it. Walking is one of the easiest, safest forms of exercise. It requires no high-powered equipment or membership in a health club. It can be done most anywhere and, in many parts of the country, year-round. Walking also takes less time overall than many other forms of exercise. After all, you need only walk out your door to get started. Unlike many sports activities, walking is something you can do solo, but it's also great to do with a friend or loved one.

Remember, too, you needn't limit yourself to one activity. If you enjoy tennis, for example, play twice a week and take a walk two or three other days. Or alternate swimming with weightlifting at your gym. Your options are limitless.

## Choose the Right Exercise for You

Not only is it important to choose an activity you enjoy, it's just as important to start out slowly. Consider any of the following low-intensity activities:

| | |
|---|---|
| Walking | Swimming |
| Bicycle riding | Yoga |
| (slow pace, on a flat | Low-impact aerobics |
| surface or exercise bicycle) | Tai chi |

If you already exercise regularly, consider "cross training."

Try one or more of the following activities to add variety to your routine:

| | |
|---|---|
| Dancing | Soccer |
| Jogging | Basketball |
| Bicycling (fast pace or | Tennis |
|   on a hilly surface) | Racquetball |
| Swimming | Squash |
| Cross-country skiing | Kick boxing, karate, |
| Using a StairMaster |   or other martial arts |

When exercising, make sure you use the proper equipment. This may be as minor an issue as digging up your swimming suit or sneakers, or as complicated as purchasing an exercise bicycle or treadmill. Whatever you do, don't let lack of equipment be your reason for inactivity. Next, find a place in your schedule to include exercise on alternate days, at least three times a week, and pencil them in. If you don't make exercise a priority, the day will be gone along with your good intentions.

## Set Exercise Goals

I've been an exerciser most of my life. I played football and basketball in high school and intramural sports in college. I've run seven marathons and countless ten-kilometer races. Like many of you, however, as I got caught up in my career and family, I began to slack off a little. One reason I did that cross-country bike trip I mentioned earlier was to set some exercise goals. For six months before that trip, I got up early a few mornings each week and cycled. I knew I'd be sorry if I weren't prepared for the trip.

Find a goal that inspires you and train to reach it. It doesn't have to be anything as ambitious as my bike trip. As I said after completing that trip, anyone who would ride a bike across the country once is determined—anyone who'd do it twice is crazy. However, a ten- to twenty-mile ride is realistic, and a lot of fun, especially if you can hook up with a bike club. Or you might try a five-kilometer walk or run. That's less than three and a half miles, and it's something most of you could do after a few months of training. Don't go into any race planning to win or set records. Just aim for your personal best and don't be discouraged by the balls of fire racing past you. Some races are charity events, so you can raise money for a good cause at the same time. Races are organized regularly in many areas, and you'll find that there's a lot of camaraderie among participants.

## Exercise With a Friend or Group

It's easy to slack off or lose motivation when you exercise by yourself, but if you've made a commitment to exercise with a friend or group, you'll be much more likely to get out there and do it. Perhaps you could get a neighbor to be your walking partner. Staying in bed for an extra few minutes is less tempting when you know someone is going to be knocking on your door for your morning walk. Furthermore, you'll find that your forty-five-minute walk will fly as you chat with your friend.

If you like tennis, racquetball, or other sports that require an opponent, set up a weekly or biweekly game through your local club. Again, if someone is counting on you to be there, you'll be there. If team sports are more your style, join a team through your health club, YMCA, or community recreation center. Consider volunteering as a referee for children's soccer or other sports leagues. These leagues are always looking for volunteers, and it's great exercise. There are lots of opportunities out there if you look for them. One summer, five of my buddies and I signed up at the local Marine base for the annual "Mud Run"—a rigorous obstacle course, complete with mud pits. We called ourselves the "Dirty Half-Dozen" and didn't come close to winning the run, but it was a blast. And it was something we all had to train for.

## Always Warm Up and Cool Down

I've asked several fitness trainers what the most common errors made by exercisers are, and they all agree. Too many people—beginners as well as conditioned athletes—fail to warm up and stretch before exercising, and they skip the cool down and stretch afterwards. If you are just beginning an exercise program, I urge you to consider exercise as a five-step routine. Make it a habit to include all five steps, which are listed below, each time you exercise.

1. *Warm up.* Whether your preferred activity is walking, bicycling, swimming, or playing tennis, the best way to prepare your body for the workout is to warm up gently. It takes only a few minutes of slow, gentle movement to gradually increase blood flow to your muscles. This allows them to relax and contract more smoothly and protects them from injury during the workout. Whether you march in place, walk on your treadmill, slowly pedal your bike, or swim a few laps, the key is to do it at an easy pace. An ideal warm-up is five to seven minutes.

2. *Stretch before the workout.* Never stretch without first warming up—a cold muscle is more prone to tearing than a warm one. When you're ready, find a comfortable surface to sit on and stretch each part of your body. (Be very careful if you have problems with your neck or back, or if you've had joint replacement surgery.) It doesn't have to be fancy. Start by extending one arm to the sky to stretch from your torso to your fingertips. Lower that arm and stretch the other side. Repeat this at least five times. Then, extend both arms, gently bend from the waist, and try to touch your toes. Never bob up and down while stretching. Simply reach as far as you can without pain, and hold the pose for ten to fifteen seconds. Again, repeat at least five times. While you stretch, breathe slowly and deeply to fill your lungs with oxygen.

3. *Exercise at a comfortable level.* One day you may be fired up and ready to go; another day you might feel the need to take it easy. Pace yourself accordingly. (Learn how to determine your target heart rate on page 134.)

4. *Cool down.* Don't go from a strenuous workout right to the sofa. As with warming up, it's important to gradually make the transition from activity to rest. Slow your pace gradually over the last few minutes of your workout, or until your heart rate returns to normal.

## Visual Scanning

The ability to scan visually is necessary for many activities, including driving a car, finding a lost object, or searching for a familiar face in a crowded room. Piecing together a jigsaw puzzle or doing some word search puzzles are two activities to help sharpen visual scanning skills.

Just for fun, try the following. Within 30 seconds, visually scan the box below and count how many times the letter E appears.

```
C F S J X E G H D S E X S D T Y Q P O M N B L E G
T H X C V R M A S B G S E Q C S E O S W T E Y B F
N S P R W H G B U N L R T V C Y U J C T Y U S W X
Q A D H S L C V P O K E T N I S C B B F V A R T H G
Z S R U O Y V R T X E B E X L S F E K Q N M E E S
D T V L K C B Y Q P W E P Z Q Y E C T B G S I O P
B L J H C B U S D Y K E E E S M T G J Q T O W S K
J H G S U E B C Y E S H N M W J L S B T L F V E S
N H M M J H E C D B V N F Y G H T X S S V T C C B
R S S T T D R U E N M K U I B R E D D K L F R C V U
Y E T T P B W A Q S T E B K X T Y Z I H T R M
```

*The letter E appears 25 times.*

5. *Stretch once more.* Stretching after your exercise routine will help prevent stiff, sore muscles the next day. Make sure one of your stretches includes reaching around and patting yourself on the back for your effort!

### Exercise at the Right Pace

When you exercise, your muscles' need for oxygenated blood increases and your heart responds by beating faster. You don't want to overdo it. Before beginning an exercise program, it is important to determine your *target heart rate*—the number of heartbeats per minute that is challenging enough to provide a good workout without putting excess strain on your heart. The steps below will help you determine your target heart rate.

### Determining Your Target Heart Rate

*For the sake of simplicity, let's assume you are a person who is fifty years old and in general good health.*

1. Begin with the number 220, which is considered to be the *theoretical* maximum heart rate at birth. It is believed that this maximum heart rate decreases by one heartbeat for every year of your life. Therefore, to determine your "personal" *maximum heart rate*, subtract your age from 220:

   $$\begin{array}{rl} 220 & \text{(maximum heart rate at birth)} \\ -\ 50 & \text{(your age)} \\ \hline 170 & \text{beats per minute (maximum heart rate)} \end{array}$$

2. To establish your *lowest* training heart rate, which is 65 percent of your maximum heart rate, multiply 170 by 65 percent:

   $$\begin{array}{rl} 170 & \text{(maximum heart rate)} \\ \times\ 0.65 & \text{(65 percent)} \\ \hline 110 & \text{beats per minute (lowest training heart rate)} \end{array}$$

3. To establish your *highest* training heart rate, which is 75 percent of your maximum heart rate, multiply 170 by 75 percent:

   $$\begin{array}{rl} 170 & \text{(maximum heart rate)} \\ \times\ 0.75 & \text{(75 percent)} \\ \hline 127 & \text{beats per minute (highest training heart rate)} \end{array}$$

This means that as a fifty-year-old who is in general good health, when exercising, your heart rate should fall between 110 and 127 beats per minute. If you are just beginning an exercise program, I recommend that you start by working slightly below your lowest heart training rate—specifically at 85 percent of this rate.

110   (lowest training heart rate)

x 0.85   (85 percent)

93   beats per minute (recommended beginning heart rate)

I recommend using this beginning rate as a target for the first two weeks of your exercise program. Then gradually work toward your low training heart rate of 110 by increasing the intensity of your workout. Because your heart will become more efficient over the weeks with regular exercise, this won't be as hard as it sounds. Eventually, you should be able to exercise without undue strain at your highest target rate of 127.

Check your heart rate five minutes into your workout, then again midway through. To measure your heart rate, first find a pulse point. Most people find it easiest to measure their pulse at the carotid arteries on either side of the neck, but you can also use your wrist. Find the pulse and count the number of beats for six seconds. (Your heart rate drops quickly the moment you stop exercising, so don't stop and count for a full minute, as you won't get an accurate reading.) Multiply the number of beats by ten and you'll have your heart rate. If you are above your target rate, slow down; if you are below it, try to move a little faster. Keep in mind that you may have lots of energy one day and little the next. Listen to your body and adjust your exercise accordingly. Don't overdo it.

### Replenish Lost Water and Nutrients

By the time you feel thirsty, you're already dehydrated. So I recommend drinking eight ounces of pure filtered water before you begin your workout, and another eight ounces afterwards. And always have a water bottle nearby. If your favorite form of exercise is walking, carry a water bottle with you so you can rehydrate on the go.

The best time to take vitamins is immediately after exercising, because physical activity primes your cells to absorb nutrients. It's also important to take vitamins with food to enhance their

# A Healthy Way to Watch TV

I don't advocate passively sitting in front of the television, but I do recommend actively working out in front of it. How do you do that? Find an exercise video geared to your interests and abilities, stick it in your VCR, clear the room of obstacles, and hit "play." Not everyone will enjoy this kind of workout, but for those who don't live near a gym, can't afford a personal trainer, or aren't comfortable exercising with a group, it could be the answer. In addition, it's a nice option to have during inclement weather or when you just don't have time to do your regular routine.

The hardest part may be selecting the right video. There are exercise videos for everything from aerobic workouts and kick boxing to dancing and yoga. The most important thing is to choose an activity you enjoy. Make sure the instructor on the tape is a certified fitness professional or has credentials in his or her field of expertise. Don't choose a video by a celebrity unless there's a certified fitness instructor either leading the class or participating in it. If possible, try a video before buying it—many libraries and video stores carry exercise videos.

Look for a tape geared to your fitness level. Most exercise videos are rated "beginner," "intermediate," and "advanced." When you outgrow one, pass it on to a friend. Check the length of the workout, which may range from twenty to ninety minutes. Workouts are carefully choreographed routines, and you'll want to complete the whole workout from warm-up to cool-down. So choose appropriately. See the Resource Section beginning on page 255 for information on purchasing workout videos.

absorption, but you don't need to sit down to a large meal—simply eating a piece of fruit will do.

## NO EXCUSES

If exercise is so good for us, why do so few Americans exercise on a regular basis? I've heard all of the excuses: "It takes too much time," "It's so boring," "It's too hard," and my personal favorite, "I'm too out of shape to exercise." Sorry, but I'm not buying any of them and neither should you. If you can make a commitment and get through the first few weeks of an exercise regimen, you will find yourself getting into the habit (you may even begin to enjoy it). Before you know it, exercise will become a habit, a habit that will provide boundless benefits for your mind, body, and spirit.

Now that we've talked about the importance of physical exercise for good memory, let's talk about the benefits of mental exercise. On to Step 6.

## STEP 6

# Sharpen Your Mind
# With Mental Workouts

*May raised six kids on a farm in Texas. After her husband died when she was in her early sixties, May continued to live alone on the farm. Although her son, who lived nearby, took over the day-to-day aspects of the farming operation, May continued to manage her own business affairs. An avid fisherman, she would load up her fishing rods and tackle into the trunk of her car and head out to the pond every chance she had, weather permitting. Although she wasn't keen on cooking (she drove into town every evening to eat dinner in a local cafeteria), she always prepared a traditional feast on Thanksgiving and Christmas for her six kids and eighteen grandchildren.*

*May was always doing something. She often visited with friends and family members, always had a jigsaw puzzle going, and routinely did the crossword puzzle and cryptogram in the daily newspaper. She read "Sports Illustrated" from cover to cover, watched professional sports on TV, and could cite the statistics of her favorite teams and players. She also played the piano beautifully and frequently—she could play almost any song by ear. May remained a lively conversationalist and engaging companion well into her eighties.*

Physical activity is but one type of exercise that benefits the brain. Among the most important things you can do to sharpen your memory and mental edge is to exercise your brain. That's right, mental workouts. Studies of older Americans reveal that those who stay involved, read, work or volunteer, spend time with friends and family, and contribute to their community are the most likely to age gracefully and stay mentally intact. Let's look at some of the people who defy the stereotype of mental aging.

Let's start with Dr. Linus Pauling. One of my heroes, Dr.

Pauling remained intensely intellectually curious and highly productive until the end of his life at age ninety-three. Although he
had won almost every honor that can be bestowed upon a scientist and humanitarian, including two Nobel prizes, he was not
one to rest on his laurels. He was almost seventy years old when
he published his groundbreaking—and establishment-shaking—
book, *Vitamin C and the Common Cold*. And he continued to pursue an enormous range of interests throughout his life. I had the
privilege of interviewing Dr. Pauling at his home on the rugged
Pacific Coast in Northern California just months before his death
in 1994. He was a gracious host, and his thoughts and words
were bright, incisive, and provocative. I asked him what he
attributed his long and productive life to, and he replied,
"Genetics plays a big part. In addition, I have always had a keen
interest in understanding more about how the world works
and in looking for opportunities to contribute. That keeps you
young."

Another example of an older person who has retained his
mental edge by embracing mental challenges is Senator John
Glenn. After making his mark on the world as one of the original
Mercury astronauts, Senator Glenn enjoyed a long and rewarding
career in the U.S. Congress. At age seventy-seven he went into
space again, thirty-six years after his first space flight. Regardless
of your opinions of politicians, I think we would all agree that
being a senator is intellectually stimulating. And space travel is a
challenge on all fronts. Senator Glenn is an excellent model of
optimal physical and mental aging.

You may know an older man or woman who inspires you
with his or her intelligence, curiosity, and insight—perhaps a parent or a family friend. You yourself might even be an inspiration
to others. What such people generally have in common is a zest
for life, curiosity, and a willingness to take on new challenges.
Whether or not they do it intentionally, these people exercise
their brains.

On the other hand, you probably also know people who have
declined mentally over the years. Not counting those with Alzheimer's disease or other forms of dementia caused by illness
or prescription drugs, I've noticed two general categories of

patients with memory and cognitive deficits—retirees and those who have recently lost a spouse.

People with busy, stimulating careers—jobs that require inter-action with others, decision making, and problem solving—tend to be quite sharp mentally. When many people retire, even if they may have been looking forward to slowing down and relaxing, they miss the contact with others and the mental stimulation. Many retirees keep themselves mentally sharp by filling this void with volunteer work, hobbies, travel, and enjoyable time with loved ones. They read books they never had the time to read before, and learn skills they'd always put off. However, those retirees who trade in their office for a couch in front of the televi-sion inevitably become bored. They are often irritable, unfocused, and physically and mentally lazy. This takes a toll on their health. Most find themselves consulting a physician for physical prob-lems. And although memory loss is rarely a primary complaint, the fact that they have become more forgetful and less focused often comes out in the course of the examination.

The other group of cognitively impaired patients I regularly encounter are those who have lost their spouses. I've seen bright, vivacious, outgoing women withdraw from the world after los-ing a spouse. Friends and neighbors reach out to them at first, but life goes on, so it seems, for everyone but them. They find that their social circle narrows—many tell me they feel like a "fifth wheel." Some, however, find renewed meaning and purpose in their lives through their children or grandchildren. Others get involved in volunteer work or even begin a new career. They make it a point to meet new people and make new friends. Yet some people—men as well as women—have a harder time. If there are no family members in their area, they may stay home alone more and have little interaction with other people. Depression to one degree or another often sets in, and they become more and more reclusive. They simply don't have enough mental stimulation. They come to my clinic, sometimes on their own but more often with a concerned loved one, prima-rily for depression, confusion, and memory loss.

These people and others suffering with memory problems and declines in mental function have been helped by following my 10-step program. And I particularly impress upon them the importance of mental exercise.

## MENTAL EXERCISE HELPS STRENGTHEN THE BRAIN

Regardless of your age, you can actually build up your brain. Like physical exercise, which creates more, stronger muscle fibers, working out your brain strengthens existing neuronal pathways and builds new nerve connections that sharpen your memory and mental edge. Let's review how these neural connections are made and then locked into your memory.

A thought, registered as a nerve impulse, travels along a neuron through its axon. Aided by neurotransmitters, the axon communicates with dendrites of other neurons across the synapses between them. The more often a thought or activity is repeated, the stronger the connections along that neural pathway become. And the more new thoughts or activities to which you are exposed, the more pathways are created in your brain.

Learning and then mastering something new actually changes your brain. Michael Merzenich, Ph.D., at the University of California at San Francisco, was involved in an experiment that vividly illustrates this point. Using a monkey as his model, he mapped out the areas of the animal's brain that were activated when it reached for food. He then trained the monkey to use only one finger to perform this task. When he again mapped the monkey's brain, he found that the area corresponding to movements of that single finger had grown by 600 percent.

Animal studies have demonstrated that intellectual challenges also cause neurons to branch out and form new connections. Marian Diamond, Ph.D., and fellow researchers at the University of California at Berkeley, have published the results of several studies comparing rats caged in a stimulating environment with toys and other rats, to those housed in smaller, ordinary cages. The animals housed in the enriched environments learned faster and were able to complete complex tasks more easily. When they were euthanized at the end of the study, their brains were found to have a 44-percent increase in dendrite branching, compared to a 21-percent increase in the animals living in the less stimulating environment. Similar studies with older animals showed that such stimulation improved mental performance in animals of any age and resulted in a thicker cerebral cortex.

Human studies have had similar results. Although both sides of the old "heredity versus environment" argument have some merit, it's been conclusively demonstrated that institutionalized infants who do not receive adequate stimulation languish, while those in an enriched environment of toys, playful interaction, and physical touch flourish, both physically and mentally. Infancy and childhood are a time of unprecedented dendrite growth and neuronal development. Neural connections are made at a rate never again experienced in one's lifetime.

Dendrite growth reaches a high point before adolescence. This is why mastering a foreign language or learning to play a musical instrument comes so much more easily to children than to adults. It's why your kids put you to shame at video games and, in many cases, anything involving a computer. Their brains simply make connections at a faster pace. After puberty, the formation of new connections slows down, and at that point the connections used frequently and repeatedly become permanent while those not used much are lost. Yet even older brains have the ability to establish new neural connections throughout life. Medical science has learned a lot about the brain in the past decade. We used to think that brain cells could not be regenerated nor new brain cells grown later in life. We now know that the brain is extremely "plastic," malleable, reparable, and able to store an almost infinite amount of new information. It just depends on how much you stimulate your brain.

In Chapter 1, I referred to the Seattle Longitudinal Study—a long-term investigation into aging. In one of the investigations, Dr. K. Warner Schaie offered men and women with declines in memory and cognitive function the opportunity to participate in five one-hour sessions that taught them how to hone their abstract reasoning skills and reaction time. After completing this course of sessions, the participants, who ranged in age from sixty-four to ninety-five, showed dramatic improvements in these areas.

## LESSONS FROM THE NUN STUDY

Dr. David Snowdon, at the University of Kentucky Sanders-Brown Center on Aging, has spearheaded a very interesting ongoing study on mental function and aging, which is funded by the National Institutes of Health. For several years now, the Nun Study has followed women belonging to the order of the School Sisters of Notre Dame, who live in a convent in Mankato, Minnesota. The sisters are an ideal study group because many of the variables that make studies like this difficult are eliminated or minimized in this tightly knit group of women. The sisters all have the same marital and reproductive histories. They engage in similar social activities and occupations, and their incomes and socioeconomic status are about the same. They have comparable diets, and none of them smoke or drink alcohol. All have access to the same medical services.

Dr. Snowdon's studies are concerned with how these women age, and particularly how their brains age. They are a remarkable group of women. They live considerably longer than the general population, and their incidence of dementia and Alzheimer's disease is minimal, even at advanced ages. Dr. Snowdon has attributed this phenomenon to their clean living (after all, they are nuns), as well as their tight social connections, shared purpose in life, and enriched environment. Beyond the lifestyle factors mentioned above, the School Sisters of Notre Dame have an ethic of intellectual stimulation. They read books, play games, work on puzzles, build their vocabularies, and contribute to the convent and community in meaningful ways throughout their lives.

But there are differences in the sisters' activities. Some are teachers while others work in less stimulating jobs. This was found to have a profound impact on their brains. In one of Dr. Snowdon's studies, brain scans showed differences in the brains of the nuns that corresponded to their level of education and job duties. Those sisters with higher education levels who taught and constantly studied and learned new information to keep up in their fields had a significantly better developed cerebral cortex, the area of the brain associated with language and reasoning. In addition, the nuns involved in less intellectually stimulating work had fewer dendrites and less branching between neurons.

Another interesting investigation in the Nun Study involved the examination of the subjects' writing samples. The sisters were required to write autobiographies just before they took their religious vows at an average age of twenty-two. The manuscripts of 107 college-educated nuns were evaluated for linguistic ability and grammatical complexity. These same nuns were tested at the ages of seventy-five to ninety-five to assess their cognitive function or, in the case of the fourteen who had died at similar ages, for Alzheimer's disease. The researchers found that "low idea density" and low grammatical complexity in the nuns' manuscripts written when they were young were associated with low cognitive test scores later in life. Of the fourteen sisters who had died, all of those whose earlier writing had low idea density (demonstrating little creativity, thought, or intellectual curiosity) had Alzheimer's disease, whereas none with high idea density did.

What this study tells us is that it's important to challenge yourself mentally throughout your life, not only in your later years. Lifelong stimulation of the brain gives it the reserves it needs to weather the inevitable changes that accompany aging, and reduces the likelihood of suffering severe mental declines in your later years.

## DESIGN A BRAIN WORKOUT PROGRAM

The exercise analogy—use it or lose it—is hard to escape. Even if you eat a perfect diet and take handfuls of nutritional supplements, you'll never be in optimal physical condition without exercise. Likewise, if you don't exercise your brain—challenge it, stimulate it, push it—it will cease to grow new connections between neurons and put you at increased risk for mental deterioration. In the remaining pages of this chapter, I'm going to offer suggestions for designing your own personal mental exercise program. Some of the activities I recommend may strike you as more physical than mental, but learning new dance steps or martial arts moves requires a great deal of cognitive activity. Other

## Television Numbs Your Mind

The average American watches thirty to fifty hours of television every week. That's over seven hours a day for some! How anyone can manage to fit in, let alone tolerate, that much TV is beyond me. Watching television is a mind-numbing activity. Even watching educational television is a passive experience that does little to stimulate your mental faculties. I understand the attraction of flaking out in front of a sitcom after a stressful day of work, but it's too easy to let TV eat up all your leisure time.

I strongly recommend that you try to eliminate or at least cut down on television watching. One immediate step you can take is to turn the TV off when you're not sitting down to watch a specific program. A television in the background is hard to ignore. It's like a magnet that draws your attention, even if you try to tune it out. The second step is to put yourself on a TV diet. You can approach this in several ways. Decide on the programs you really want to watch and turn the TV off when they're over. Or ration your time in front of the TV to, say, one hour a day. Another option is to limit the types of shows you watch—the news, perhaps, or an occasional movie or history program. Like any diet, you may feel deprived at first, but you will be doing yourself and your family an enormous favor by turning off the "boob-tube."

suggestions, like listening to music, may seem passive and appear to involve no learning at all. However, as I will show you, certain types of music actually stimulate the brain.

The good thing about mental workouts is that they're fun. While the initiation of a physical fitness program is often accompanied by sore muscles and possibly a certain amount of pain, these mental exercises are nothing but enjoyable. Think back to your childhood when you spent hours involved in a good book or a spirited game of Monopoly, checkers, or cards. This state of relaxed concentration is what we're aiming for. It's important that you approach these brain workouts in a systematic manner. Decide which ones suit you and set aside a place in your schedule for them several times a week. Plan for it and make it happen. Go for variety. The more you repeat a certain exercise or activity, the easier it becomes, so try a combination of the following mental challenges.

## Read

Reading is a great way to challenge your mind. Of course, it's great to read newspapers, light novels, and magazines, but make sure you also read things that stimulate your brain. I am an avid reader. To keep up in medicine I have to read stacks of medical journals and books. But I also like to have another book or two going. Some of the books I've enjoyed in the last year are *A Civil Action*, Jonathan Harr's stirring true story of a lawsuit filed by the families of leukemia victims against an industrial giant; Tom Wolfe's *A Man in Full* (a novel set in my hometown, Atlanta, Georgia); Harry Dent's *The Roaring 2000s*, a fascinating look at social and economic trends making their way into the new millennium; and *Into Thin Air: A Personal Account of the Mount Everest Disaster* by Jon Krakauer.

I also enjoy rereading some of the classics. You'd be surprised at how much better these timeless tales are once you have a little maturity and insight (not to mention that now you don't *have* to read them for English class). If you're a fiction reader, delve into nonfiction—a biography or a subject that has always interested you. Treat it as a study course and really learn what you're reading. If you generally read more serious nonfiction, lighten up with a good novel and tune into the style and language of the story.

## Get Hooked on Books on Audiotape and Educational Tapes

Nothing makes a repetitive, boring activity like driving long distances more fun than popping an interesting cassette into your car's tape player. I'm hooked on books on audiotape. I drive thirty to forty-five minutes each way from home to my office, and rather than flip through the radio stations trying to find something of interest among the inane blather and top-40 music, I put in a tape. With a good book or lecture going, I'm never in a hurry.

I even drive the speed limit (a rarity in Southern California). Sometimes I'll actually stay in the car in the parking lot to listen to the end of a chapter or section.

You can check out tapes from your library, purchase them in bookstores, or rent them. A number of mail order companies rent and sell books on audiotape (many unabridged) for reasonable prices. Some also provide wonderful educational tapes on a wide variety of subjects, from health issues and political discussions to all manners of self-improvement courses. See the Resource Section beginning on page 255 for more information.

## Listen to Music

You know that music can lift your mood and calm your stress, but can listening to music increase your IQ? Evidence points in that direction. Gordon Shaw, Ph.D., and other researchers at the University of California in Irvine, studied the effects of music on the IQs of thirty-six students. After their baseline IQs had been determined, the students either listened to Mozart's *Sonata for Two Pianos in D Major, K. 448;* did a relaxation exercise; or just sat quietly. They were then retested. The researchers discovered that listening to music temporarily raised the students' IQs by an average of nine points. After listening to Mozart, their average IQ was 119, compared to 111 after the relaxation exercise, and 110 with silence. Dr. Shaw postulated that the complexity of Mozart's themes and rhythms might somehow open up or facilitate the electrical pathways in the brain involved in critical thinking and problem solving. The "Mozart Effect" has been examined in other studies, and this music has been observed to modify EEG activity in the frontal and temporal regions of the brain, which are involved in problem solving and memory.

The effects of other types of music on cognitive function have also been investigated. In a 1998 study involving 144 adults and teenagers, researchers from the Institute of HeartMath in Boulder Creek, California, examined how various types of music affected listeners' tension level, mood, and mental clarity. They compared four kinds of music: grunge rock, classical, new age, and "designer" music that had been created specifically for the study. Grunge rock produced overall negative effects on mood and cognition in everyone tested, even those teenagers who liked the music. Classical and new age music produced mixed, overall neutral results, while the designer music resulted in enhancements in mood and mental clarity.

My house is alive with music—sometimes *too* alive in a household of teenagers with several different types of music going at the same time. My personal tastes vary from '50s rock and roll to opera to the score from *Les Miserables.* But when I'm writing and working, I take a lesson from the Mozart study and play classical music softly in the background.

## Play Games and Solve Puzzles

According to Dr. Gene Cohen, former director of the National Institutes of Health, Center on Aging, "Games . . . really fun, captivating games are the mental counterpart to physical exercise. If you can work up a mental sweat doing something that is also fun, you've tingled your brain cells in a way they won't forget." I couldn't agree more. Some of our happiest family times are spent playing games. When my children were very young, they loved the board game Candyland. I got so tired of playing it that I'd cheat to let them win. However, there are many great games not geared for three-years-olds that are fun and really make you think. Games like chess, bridge, and a number of other card games involve complex strategy. Other games like Scrabble, Trivial Pursuit, and Scattergories stimulate your memory and force you to dredge things out of your deepest memory banks. MindTrap, which is a game of brain teasers, taps into your creativity and problem-solving skills. These games not only exercise your mind, they also require spirited social interaction, which itself is good for mental health. More solitary pursuits, such as jigsaw puzzles, cryptograms, crossword puzzles, brainteasers, and math games, are also fun and stimulating. Check out a game or toy store, library, or bookstore for more ideas. You'll be surprised at how many fun, challenging mental exercises await you.

Also, don't make the mistake of thinking video games are just for kids. They have become incredibly sophisticated in the last

# Classic Brain Teasers

Try these classic brain teasers to give your brain a little mental exercise.

1. Is there a fourth of July in England?
2. Why can't a man living in Miami be buried west of the Mississippi River?
3. How many birthdays does the average man have?
4. If a doctor gave you three pills and told you to take one every half hour, how long would the pills last you?
5. A farmer has twenty-six sheep. All but nine die. How many does he have left?
6. An archeologist finds a coin dated "46 BC." Why does he think it isn't authentic?
7. A woman gives a beggar a dollar. The woman is the beggar's sister, but the beggar is not the woman's brother. How can this be?
8. What goes up and down but doesn't move?
9. What can go up a chimney down, but can't go down a chimney up?
10. This one is just for fun. You can wow your friends with it.

   - Pick a number between 1 and 9.
   - Multiply that number by 9.
   - Subtract 5.
   - If the number is two digits, add the digits together. If the number is still two digits, add the digits again (eg., If your number is 64, add 6 + 4 = 10. Then add 1 + 0 = 1).
   - Match the number to a corresponding letter of the alphabet (1=A, 2=B, 3=C, 4=D, etc.).
   - Think of a country in Europe that begins with that letter.
   - Take the second letter in the country name and think of an animal that begins with that letter.
   - What color is that animal?

*Turn to page 152 for the answers.*

few years. I even got hooked on one called Tetris, which involves manipulating the arrangement of falling bricks in order to stack them into a solid wall. The worst of it is I still can't beat those darned kids!

## Memorize

Socrates tells a story about the creation of writing. One of the Egyptian gods shows his invention to another god who voices his disapproval. "This discovery of yours will create forgetfulness in the learners' souls, because they will not use their memories; they will trust to the external written characters and not remember themselves." I'm sure many of you, like me, had to do a lot of memorization in school—poems, passages from famous speeches, and the like. I can remember to this day the opening lines of Lincoln's Gettysburg Address, the Declaration of Independence, and several Shakespearean passages, even though I've rarely thought of them over the years.

Memorization has all but disappeared from most current curricula, to the detriment of today's students, in my opinion. Memorization is an intense mental exercise. Pull out a favorite poem or passage you find especially meaningful and take the time and effort to memorize it.

## Learn a New Word Every Day

Set a goal to learn one new vocabulary word every day. When you come across a word you're unfamiliar with in your reading, take a minute or two to look it up. Take note of the origin of the word—it is often fascinating and will help you remember it. I always keep a dictionary near my desk (it's one of those ten-pound monsters). Once you learn a new word, you'll be surprised at how often it pops up in print and conversation. Browsing a thesaurus is another way to pick up new words, as is reading the *Reader's Digest* vocabulary section and calendars that highlight a new word every day. If you are on the Internet regularly, you might consider subscribing to Merriam-Webster's Word of the Day mailing list. You'll get a new word via e-mail every day. To subscribe online, visit Merriam-Webster's website (http://www.m-w.com/service/subinst.htm).

## Write

History would be not be as rich without the letters of Thomas Jefferson and John Adams, Napoleon and Josephine, Vincent Van Gogh and his brother Theo, and many others. The personal letters of historical figures give us great insight into their humanity, and the letters of more common folks provide us with a window into history. Now that it's so easy and inexpensive to pick up a telephone, letter writing has become something of a lost art. Yet the process of sitting down, focusing your mind, and putting your thoughts down on paper is an excellent mental exercise. In addition to giving your brain a workout, letters strengthen social and family relationships. Phone calls are nice, but getting a personal

---

### ANSWERS TO CLASSIC BRAIN TEASERS ON PAGE 150:

1. Yes, but it isn't celebrated as Independence Day.
2. If he's living, he can't be buried.
3. Only one—you can be born only once.
4. The pills would last for one hour—you would take one pill immediately, the second one 30 minutes later, and the third pill 30 minutes after that.
5. Nine—that's how many were left.
6. How would the ancients know they were living 46 years "Before Christ"?
7. The beggar is the woman's sister.
8. The temperature.
9. An umbrella.
10. Gray. No matter which number you choose in the first step, you will always end up with the number 4, which corresponds to the letter "D." *Most* people pick "Denmark" as the country that begins with "D." And *most* people pick "elephant" for an animal that begins with the letter "E." And elephants are gray.

letter in the mail is a treat for anyone, and letters are often treasured by their recipients. I wouldn't be surprised if most of you have at least one special letter squirreled away somewhere.

Letters aside, writing is an excellent mental discipline. Consider keeping a journal or trying your hand at letters to the editor of your local paper. Try writing a story, a poem, or an article. You might discover that you have a knack for it and decide to pursue writing in a more serious manner. But even if you're just writing for yourself, it's an endeavor I highly recommend.

## Master New Knowledge

Decide on a subject you're interested in and learn everything you can about it. Get out the encyclopedia, surf the Internet, and search the library or bookstore for information on the subject. Attend lectures, take a class at a local college or community center, listen to a taped instruction series, or hire a tutor. Your choices here are limited only by your imagination.

You might decide to learn a foreign language, something that really stretches the brains of adults. If you're interested in travel, learn all you can about the places you'd like to visit. If health issues are your cup of tea, look into the lecture series offered by healthcare facilities. Those of you interested in political or community issues might want to attend local and state government meetings and see how things are really run. Your research will lead you down unexpectedly interesting paths and may even open up new worlds.

## Acquire New Skills

So far, we've talked mostly about verbal and analytical learning, but another great way to stimulate your brain is by doing. Learn to play a musical instrument. Give ballroom dancing or square dancing a try. Indulge in art lessons. Take up martial arts or yoga. Learn to bowl, sail a boat, or fly fish. Try your hand at knitting, pottery making, embroidery, or woodworking. Last year we got a pool table for our rec room, and I decided I wanted to get good at the game. I had shot a little pool in high school and college but never had the time to play much. Once I had the table at home, I figured it would be a good opportunity to improve my skills. I took a few lessons and quickly learned that pool is a much more cerebral game than most people give it credit for. Now, you'd better watch out for me if we ever meet up in a pool hall!

More recently, I've taken up trapshooting and skeet shooting. In these sports, targets called clay pigeons are thrown into the air. You track them and shoot them with a shotgun. It's a lot of fun

## Exercises to Stimulate Creative Thinking

Try the following exercises, which stimulate the areas of the brain involved in creative thinking. These same thought processes are involved in brainstorming—from which many of our best ideas come. Although you can try these exercises alone, competing with someone else makes it more of a game.

1. List as many synonyms as you can for the word "fast." Try this with other common words, such as "slow," "run," and "talk."

2. How many ways can you complete the following sentences?

   • It is as big as _____.

   • He is as smart as_____.

   • It is as small as _____.

   • She is as pretty as_____.

3. Write each letter of the alphabet on a piece of paper, one letter per line. As quickly as you can, list an animal that begins with each letter. Do this again with kinds of foods, articles of clothing, men's and women's names, and any other category you can think of.

4. List every word you can think of that begins with the letter "I" (or any other letter) within three minutes.

5. Name every type of flower you can think of, or dog breeds, desserts, card games, etc.

and quite competitive. These are actually Olympic sports, and I've developed a real passion for them. I've gotten involved at a local club, and one of my sons often accompanies me, which makes it even more fun. The point is that it's never too late to teach an old dog new tricks, and who knows? Grandma Moses, one of American's most beloved artists, didn't take up painting until her seventies.

## Stretch Your Imagination

Daydream. Have a mental conversation with Abraham Lincoln or Pablo Picasso—ask questions and imagine how they would respond. Try to remember your nighttime dreams. Go skiing or surfing or rock climbing—in your mind. Challenge yourself to a memory marathon. Visualize the house you grew up in and take yourself on a guided tour in your mind. How was your room decorated when you were a child? What did the kitchen smell like? What pictures were on the walls? Or choose a day in your past of some importance, your wedding day, for example. Relive that day in vivid detail. Who was there? Picture what you and your spouse were wearing, the decorations, the food. Try to recapture your feelings. Spend time and flesh out the details in each of these exercises, and when your mind wanders, rein it back in.

This kind of activity may seem silly and will be especially challenging for you "left-brained" analytical people. But using your imagination like this stimulates creativity and gives your brain a workout.

## Get Involved and Give of Yourself

Social interaction nourishes the brain. Notice how many of the suggestions in this section require being with other people or getting out in the world? Simply conversing with others is mentally stimulating. It is important to maintain strong social relationships. Meet new people. Invite old friends to share new activities. Visit museums, go to movies, or read the same book and then discuss it. Getting involved in the flow of life is especially important if you live alone. There are so many volunteer opportunities out there. Hospitals, nursing homes, preschools, churches, scout troops, homeless shelters, soup kitchens—these are all possibilities for you to give your most valuable assets, your time and your heart.

Jack, a retired professor in his late sixties, has become a "baby holder." Twice a week for several hours Jack goes to the neonatal care unit in the local hospital where premature babies and ill newborns stay, sometimes for weeks or months. Because their stays are so long, their families aren't able to be there all the time, and as much as they need medical care, these babies also need a warm, loving body to hold and rock them. Jack gets a lot of kudos for this volunteer work, but he says that it is more gratifying to him than it could possibly be to the babies.

## SUMMING IT UP

Mental workouts—exercises for your brain—are both easy and fun. And, as you have seen in this step, there are scores of different ways to exercise your brain. And all will help keep you sharp. In addition to the benefits described, all brain-building exercises have one additional benefit. They help reduce stress, which has detrimental effects on your brain and contributes to memory loss and mental declines. In Step 7, you'll see exactly how stress affects your brain, and learn some simple solutions for managing it.

( **STEP 7** )

# Reduce
# Mind-Numbing Stress

*M*aggie, *a fifty-year-old mother of three teenagers, works in a high-stress job in the publishing industry. It is one of those jobs that require constant juggling of several projects at once and jumping from deadline to deadline. As a rule, she handles it well and thrives on the excitement. However, after two months of particularly arduous deadlines and nonstop work, Maggie came to see me with concerns about her memory. She related a nightmare of a business trip she had just taken. It began at the airport where she discovered that she had forgotten her driver's license. She was able to get on her flight only after her husband faxed a copy of her license to the airline. Over the next few days, she lost her purse in the parking lot of her hotel, left her planner in a conference room, misplaced her car keys twice, and just before an important presentation, realized that she had forgotten to bring a vital document with her. Maggie was sure she was losing it.*

I see too many patients like Maggie. Although the details of each of their busy lives are unique, they're all buckling under the weight of chronic stress. Anything you find physically or mentally threatening or upsetting causes stress. As such, stress is extremely subjective. What is perceived as stressful to you may be "just one of those things" to someone else. For example, I hate waiting in lines. I find myself growing impatient, eyeing the faster moving lines, and feeling irritated when my line refuses to budge. Yet I know that many others just bide their time and don't let the wait bother them. On the other hand, I find deadlines, which simply overwhelm a lot of people, invigorating. In fact, I do most of my best work under the pressure of time constraints.

But regardless of what it is that gets you worked up, the body's reaction is universal. Technically, this is termed the *gener-*

*al adaptation syndrome,* but more often it is called the *stress response.* It is a carryover of the physiological and biochemical changes that launched our ancestors into action and saved their lives and limbs from the physical dangers of their world.

The stress response begins with a perceived threat. Your senses send an alarm message to your brain—specifically to the thalamus, through the limbic system to the hypothalamus and pituitary gland. The pituitary releases a hormone that activates the adrenal glands, which in turn secrete the "stress" hormones epinephrine (also called adrenaline) and norepinephrine (also called noradrenaline). These hormones quickly flood your tissues and initiate a series of physiological changes. Your heart and respiration rates increase, and your blood vessels constrict, directing blood flow to your muscles. Digestion slows down as blood is shunted away from the stomach. Blood sugar elevates to give you a burst of energy. Your brain is bathed in norepinephrine and other chemicals that make you more alert and responsive. You might feel excited, afraid, flushed or have a butterflies-in-the-stomach sensation.

This is the *alarm reaction* phase of the stress response, and it is indispensable when you are faced with physical danger. It makes you run faster and fight harder, which is why it is often called the "fight-or-flight" response. Once the danger has passed, hormone levels subside and things return to normal. However, if the perception of threat persists, a second stage in the stress response known as the *resistance reaction* sets in. And this is when stress becomes a problem. Additional adrenal hormones called glucocorticoids or corticosteroids (which include cortisol) are churned out, and other chemical changes occur as the body prepares to dig in and remain in the "full alert" mode. Protein is converted to energy, blood pressure elevates, and magnesium, potassium, and other nutrients are depleted. The final stage of the stress response is *exhaustion.* Adrenal hormone stores are depleted, and organ systems begin to fail. For a summary of the general adaptation syndrome, see Table 4.2.

The exhaustion phase is rare; however, many people get stuck in the resistance phase of the stress response. This happens because our bodies, based on eons of evolution, are still programmed to react to perceived threats with a physical response. Of course, we can intellectually differentiate between physical threats that require action, and emotional or psychological threats that are more appropriately handled in other ways—but our bodies cannot. So we have to go through this whole rigma-role every time we feel threatened. For some people, this happens many times during the day, and it results in what we call *chronic*

## TABLE 4.2. THE GENERAL ADAPTATION SYNDROME (STRESS RESPONSE)

As the following table clearly shows, chronic stress forces your body to soak in a veritable soup of adrenal chemicals. Research has linked chronic stress to a wide variety of health conditions, including anxiety disorders, depression, and memory loss.

| Alarm Reaction Phase | Resistance Reaction Phase | Exhaustion Phase |
|---|---|---|
| • Adrenocorticotropic hormone (ACTH) released by pituitary gland. | • Cortisol and other corticosteroids secreted by adrenal cortex. | • Glucocorticoid stores are depleted. |
| • Epinephrine and norepinephrine released by the adrenal medulla. | • Conversion of protein to energy. | • Hypoglycemia. |
| • Heart rate increases. | • Sodium retention to elevate blood pressure. | • Potassium ion loss. |
| • Blood and oxygen diverted to muscles and brain. | • Subconscious coping behavior. | • Collapse of specific organs. |
| • Sweat increases to eliminate toxins and lower body temperature. |  | • Total collapse of body function. |
| • Blood sugar increases. |  |  |
| • Liver delivers stored glucose into bloodstream. |  |  |

*stress.* Chronic stress contributes to a host of health problems, including muscular tension, digestive difficulties, and elevated blood pressure. But one of the areas hit hardest by chronic stress is your brain.

## HOW STRESS AFFECTS YOUR BRAIN

During the initial stage of stress, norepinephrine makes your mind alert and perceptive. This is "good stress." It motivates and keeps you focused. It may cause you to feel a little nervous, but overall you think clearly and your memory is sharper than ever. The resistance phase of the stress response, however, is bad news. Prolonged exposure to cortisol and other glucocorticoids has a decidedly negative effect on your brain. These hormones generate free radicals, which damage neurons and impair cognitive function. And unlike norepinephrine, which subsides after things have quieted down, these hormones remain in your system for hours.

This may explain why some students, even if they've studied hard, do poorly on examinations. Or why you can spend days preparing a speech, but when you get up in front of an audience, your mind goes blank. The stress you've been under messes with your memory. It has long been known that glucocorticoids interfere with the transfer of short-term memories into long-term memory storage. Researchers at the Center for the Neurobiology of Learning and Memory, at the University of California at Irvine, have discovered that these stress hormones also affect information retrieval and recall. As Benno Roozendaal, coauthor of this recent study, states, "If you are in a stressful situation, it's not important to remember things like two plus two equals four—the most important thing is to run away."

The chronic stress we often find ourselves under means that these hormones remain dangerously elevated. High levels of cortisol are clearly associated with atrophy of the hippocampus, the area of the brain that processes memory. And older people with high levels of this stress hormone often have memory impairment. A 1998 study published in *Nature Neuroscience* involved fifty-one healthy older individuals who were followed for five or six years. During that time, their cortisol levels were measured, and they were given periodic tests to gauge their memory and cognitive function. It was found that the subjects with high and increasing cortisol levels had a 14-percent decrease in hippocampal volume, based on MRI studies. They also had problems with delayed recall, and it took them longer to follow steps on tests of cognitive function. The researchers concluded that "long-term exposure to adrenal stress hormones may promote hippocampal aging in normal elderly humans," and "chronic stress may accelerate hippocampal deterioration."

Stress is often accompanied by depression and anxiety, which in and of themselves may cause memory problems. The frequency of these conditions increases with age. The aging brain is more susceptible to biochemical imbalances, and the elderly are also more likely to be faced with events in their lives that trigger anxiety and depression—deaths of loved ones, financial difficulties, illness, and the like. Both depression and anxiety increase the likelihood of the filtering errors discussed in the first chapter. When you are besieged by worry or anxiety, it's hard to focus your attention. You may forget things because they never made it into long-term memory—there were simply too many competing stimuli. Stress and sleep disturbances also often go hand in hand, and inadequate sleep affects your memory and ability to function at your mental peak.

## REDUCE STRESS AND SHARPEN YOUR MENTAL EDGE

Now that you know how stress affects your brain and cognitive function, let's get to the crux of the matter. What can you do about this problem? This step of the program offers a number of suggestions for dealing with stress. However, if severe stress, depression, or anxiety is overwhelming and interfering with your state of mind and health, please consult a medical professional.

One point I've tried to make clear in this book is that our minds and bodies are an integrated whole. Although some therapies target specific conditions (such as the herbs and smart drugs that help improve memory and mental edge), most suggested therapies that promote the health and healing of one part of your

## Social Readjustment Scale

To some degree, stress is subjective. What one person might consider stressful, another person may take in stride. There are, however, certain events that typically create stress in most people. Use the following scale to assess your personal stress level. If your points total 200 or more, stress may be a contributing factor to any memory problem you may be experiencing.

| Rank | Life Event | Mean Value |
|------|------------|-----------|
| 1. | Death of a spouse | 100 |
| 2. | Divorce | 73 |
| 3. | Marital separation | 65 |
| 4. | Jail or prison term | 63 |
| 5. | Death of close family member | 63 |
| 6. | Personal injury or illness | 53 |
| 7. | Getting married | 50 |
| 8. | Getting fired | 47 |
| 9. | Marital reconciliation | 45 |
| 10. | Retirement | 45 |
| 11. | Illness of a family member | 44 |
| 12. | Pregnancy | 40 |
| 13. | Sexual difficulties | 39 |
| 14. | Gain of new family member | 39 |
| 15. | Business adjustment | 39 |
| 16. | Change in financial status | 38 |
| 17. | Death of a close friend | 37 |

body are beneficial for overall good health. For example, foods that protect against heart disease also reduce the risk of diabetes. Vitamins and minerals protect cells throughout your body, and exercise strengthens virtually all of your body's systems. In a similar vein, many of the recommendations in this program for sharpening memory are also great stress busters. Let's briefly review them.

| | | |
|---|---|---|
| 18. | Change to a new line of work | 36 |
| 19. | Increased arguments with spouse | 35 |
| 20. | A large mortgage | 31 |
| 21. | Foreclosure of mortgage or loan | 30 |
| 22. | Change in work responsibilities | 29 |
| 23. | Child leaving home | 29 |
| 24. | Trouble with in-laws | 29 |
| 25. | Outstanding personal achievement | 28 |
| 26. | Spouse beginning or stopping job | 26 |
| 27. | Beginning or ending school | 26 |
| 28. | Change in living conditions | 25 |
| 29. | Change in personal habits | 24 |
| 30. | Trouble with boss | 23 |
| 31. | Change in work hours or conditions | 20 |
| 32. | Change in residence | 20 |
| 33. | Change in school | 20 |
| 34. | Change in recreational activities | 19 |
| 35. | Change in church activities | 19 |
| 36. | Change in social activities | 18 |
| 37. | Small mortgage | 17 |
| 38. | Change in sleeping habits | 16 |
| 39. | Change in number of family get-togethers | 15 |
| 40. | Change in eating habits | 15 |
| 41. | Preparing for vacation | 15 |
| 42. | Christmas (or other busy holiday season) | 12 |
| 43. | Minor problems with the law | 11 |

**Total Score** _____

## Eat Right for Less Stress

The diet described in Step 1 of the program will go a long way toward keeping you on an emotionally even keel. Low-glycemic carbohydrates, such as vegetables and fruits, prevent blood sugar fluctuations that leave some people irritable and moody. Lean protein from fish, skinless poultry, low-fat or nonfat dairy products, and beans and legumes provide the stamina you need to function at your best. And avoidance of dietary disasters that have virtually no nutritional value—fatty animal products, refined carbohydrates, hydrogenated fats, and processed oils— improves overall health and spares your reserves so you can function at your best.

## Avoid Caffeine

I particularly recommend that you avoid caffeine. As explained in Step 1, you may think caffeine makes you more alert, but it really doesn't. What caffeine actually does is set off a stress response. It stimulates your adrenal glands to make epinephrine and norepinephrine—the same stress hormones that are pro- duced in response to any stressor. This sets the stress response in motion, causing tense muscles, elevated blood sugar, and in- creased pulse and respiration. You may feel mentally sharper because your brain is high on adrenaline. It's ready to rumble. One cup of coffee for most people isn't damaging. But as you may recall from our discussion of the three stages of the stress response, if stress hormones remain elevated, the body is thrown into a state of chronic stress. By sipping on coffee, tea, or caf- feinated soda all day long, you are forcing your adrenal glands to continue to pump out stress hormones.

One of the simplest steps you can take to reduce your level of stress is to cut back on caffeine to no more than one cup of coffee a day. Replace it with a cup of green tea, which has considerably less caffeine and a host of cancer-fighting phytochemicals. Better yet, eliminate caffeine entirely. It may be difficult at first, especially if you're a big coffee drinker. You may experience headaches, edgi- ness, and even lack of focus and concentration at first. Getting off caffeine is like withdrawing from any addictive drug. But if you can live with these symptoms for a few days, you'll find over the course of the next few weeks that you are calmer, clearer minded, and less nervous than you were when you were consuming caf- feine. You'll be thankful that you've lost the coffee "crutch." I'll never forget a fishing trip I took with a friend many years ago. There we were in the pristine wilderness with nothing but God's majesty for miles around us. Yet this man was miserable. All he could think about was that he'd forgotten to bring coffee.

### Replenish Lost Nutrients

Stress zaps your body of nutrients. One of the most significant of these losses is magnesium, a mineral required in hundreds of biochemical interactions. Very low magnesium levels affect the brain and may result in confusion and other signs of cognitive dysfunction. Another mineral deficiency caused by stress is in potassium, which the body loses in an effort to hang onto sodium. B-complex vitamins are also eaten up when your body is suffering from chronic stress. Many of the B vitamins are important for the proper functioning of the brain and nervous system, and deficiencies can cause memory loss and, in some cases, severe dementia. Because free radicals are also produced during stress, antioxidant stores are depleted. By replacing these lost nutrients, you will help your body combat the ill effects of stress. A high-dose multivitamin and mineral supplement offers you the best protection. (For a listing of recommended daily nutrients, see Table 4.1 on page 100.)

### Exercise

Vigorous physical exercise stimulates the production of endorphins, your body's "feel-good" neurotransmitters. But even less intense physical activity reduces stress. Walking in the park, working in your garden, bowling with friends—all of these activities (none of which would be considered particularly strenuous) improve your mood and lighten your soul. In Step 5, I explained some of the nuts and bolts of exercise, how to get started, ways to motivate yourself, and precautions you should take. If you put aside the time for a few exercise sessions in your busy schedule each week, that step alone—making time for yourself and your own needs—is a powerful stress-reduction tool.

### Take a Stress Vacation With Mental Exercise

I discussed a number of activities that work out your brain in Step

6. While you might find the concept of mental exercise tiring, you'll find that taking a little time out to play a game, solve a puzzle, or read a book can be surprisingly relaxing—and a lot of fun. These activities demand focused attention. You are required to take leave of your problems for the duration and shift your attention elsewhere. Spending time with others and giving of yourself requires a similar effort. It allows you to get a handle on stress while helping others at the same time. Getting into the flow of life is one of the most powerful of all stress reducers.

## Tune in to Music

One of the simplest ways of reducing stress is listening to music. Clinical studies have shown that listening to music decreases blood pressure and heart rate and modifies stress hormone levels. Music can work its de-stressing magic even if it is played in the background. I bring my favorite classical CDs into the office and play them while I work. The type of music you choose to listen to depends on your personal tastes, but I guarantee that you can find some kind of music to foster peace and relaxation.

## Get Plenty of Sleep

Although most of us don't give it much thought (we sleep right through it), sleep is an incredibly important event, especially for your brain. When you sleep, your brain discharges, getting ready for the next day's onslaught of stimuli. Optimal mental and emotional function require a well-rested brain, and feeling upbeat and in control is just about impossible when you don't get enough sleep. If you're having problems sleeping, or just don't manage to get enough sleep, it is important that you make a concerted effort to catch up on your "sleep debt." In Step 8, you'll learn how to get a good night's sleep, for sleep is an important stress reducer.

## Take Hormones That Combat Stress

Melatonin and DHEA are two hormones that counter the negative effects of stress. As explained in Step 8, melatonin facilitates sleep. It also buffers the harmful effects of cortisol and other corticosteroids on the brain, and increases the production of endorphins, the "feel-good" neurotransmitters that relieve pain and elevate mood.

DHEA, which is discussed in detail in Step 9, is inversely related to stress hormone levels—as levels of corticosteroids rise, DHEA levels fall. Therefore, if you are under a lot of stress and your adrenal glands are kicking out a lot of stress hormones, it is likely that your DHEA levels are low. And this can hamper your body's ability to withstand the effects of stress. Supplemental DHEA has been demonstrated in a number of animal studies to improve resistance to stress. Animals supplemented with DHEA were able to endure a number of stressors—including temperature extremes, extended physical exercise, chemical toxins, and microbial agents—that injured, sickened, or even killed animals not given DHEA.

### Get Control of Your Time

Maggie, whose story I shared with you in the opening of this chapter, was having significant memory problems that were affecting her job performance and her personal life. I put my finger on Maggie's problem right away—she was just too darn busy. She commuted an hour to work every day, worked nine or ten hours, then rushed home to more of the same—cooking, laundry, kids' homework, and her own catch-up work. She fell into bed at midnight, woke up at 5:30, and did it all over again. I placed her on my 10-step program and strongly advised her to take control of her time.

Taking my advice, Maggie looked hard at her schedule and saw that she was able to carve out a few hours a week for herself. She learned how to make lists and prioritize her activities. She enlisted her family's support, and they began to pitch in more around the house. One of the most important things Maggie learned was how to say "no" and to be realistic about how much work and responsibility she takes on. She's still busy. She still spends a lot of time at work and most of her leisure time with her husband and children, but for the first time, she feels she is in control of her daily schedule. And as a result, she feels less stressed and more clearheaded.

Listen to the advice of poet Carl Sandburg in the following words:

> *Time is the coin of your life. It is the only coin you have,*
> *and only you can determine how it will be spent.*
> *Be careful lest you let other people spend it for you.*

## De-Stress With Your Breath

Earlier in this chapter, I described the stress response in terms of what happens inside your body, in your muscles, glands, and bloodstream. These are things over which you have little control. However, there is one aspect of the stress response that you can control—your breathing. As stress hormones cause your heart to pump faster to deliver more blood and oxygen to your muscles, your breathing also changes, going from slow and deep to rapid and shallow. Your body is preparing for action, and your breath is quickening in anticipation.

An easy way to interrupt the stress response—and one that you can do anytime and anywhere—is to consciously slow your breathing. Inhale slowly, hold the breath for a few seconds, then exhale slowly. Try it: Inhale, two, three, four. Hold, two, three, four. Exhale, two, three, four. Repeat this three or four times. Once your breath normalizes, your body will follow. It may not "hear" you right away, but if you continue to breathe slowly and deeply, your brain and body will get the message and calm down. Instead of churning out more stress chemicals and setting you up for chronic stress, your body will learn a much healthier relaxation response. Your heart rate will slow, your blood pressure will drop, and less easily measured signs of stress will also abate.

For many people, combining slow, deep breathing with the mental repetition of a word is easier than focusing on the breath itself. Choose a word that you find soothing ("love," "God," or "peace" are common choices) and mentally repeat it with each inhalation and exhalation. The silent repetition of a word pulls your attention away from the alarm bells going off in your body and frantic thoughts running through your mind. You pass from the hyperalertness of stress to the alertness of focused attention to a state of relaxation and peacefulness.

## Employ Progressive Relaxation Techniques

Ever notice how tense your muscles get when you're stressed? It's a natural part of the fight-or-flight response. Not surprisingly, muscular tension is physically and mentally exhausting. A great technique for untying the knots of stress is progressive relaxation. Simply sit in a comfortable chair or lie down in a comfortable position. Consciously tense every muscle in your body—your facial muscles, neck, shoulders, arms, wrists, hands, stomach, buttocks, thighs, calves, ankles, and feet. Then let them go all at once. Feel the difference? Your breath should become slower and more relaxed when you release the muscular tension in your body.

Now, starting at your toes and working upward slowly, consciously relax each muscle in your body, one at a time. Each of us tends to hold tension in a certain part of the body. It might be your back or stomach, shoulders or face—so consciously relax each body part as you work your way to the crown of your head. When you're finished, your muscles should be completely relaxed. Sit or lie still for a few minutes, focusing on your breathing or silently repeating your soothing word. When you're ready, move slowly into your next activity.

Whether you focus on your breath or let go of muscular tension in your body, relaxation techniques such as these can result in dramatic improvements in markers of stress. Deep relaxation causes oxygen consumption to drop by about 12 percent almost immediately—a drop similar to that experienced during sleep. In addition, blood lactate levels, which build up with anxiety, decrease by up to 20 percent. You can practice these relaxation techniques at regular times throughout the day, or use them when you feel stressed. Either way, you will be protecting your body and brain from the negative effects of stress.

## Take Stress-Reducing Herbs

A number of herbs contain stress-reducing properties. The most well known are ginseng, St. John's wort, and kava.

### Ginseng

Ginseng is a medicinal herb that has been used for thousands of years for its healing properties. It helps memory and cognitive function by modulating the harmful effects of stress. As such, it is classified as an *adaptogen,* a term coined in 1957 by Russian scientist Dr. I. Brekhman. It denotes substances that improve the body's ability to adapt to a broad range of physical and biochemical stressors.

Ginseng is an exceptionally adaptable plant. It has been around for million of years, enduring the Ice Age and other climactic extremes that have wiped out many plant and animal species. The most widely used type of ginseng is Korean ginseng (*Panax ginseng,* which means all-healing or panacea in Greek). *Panax ginseng* is used in traditional Chinese medicine to enhance stamina and the capacity to cope with fatigue and stress. It is also used as a tonic for its revitalizing properties, especially after a long illness.

The source of *Panax ginseng's* adaptogenic properties are phytochemicals called *ginsenosides.* These help balance the hypothalamus, as well as the pituitary and adrendal glands, which are involved in the stress response. Ginsenosides have been shown to prevent free-radical damage and to enhance the immune response. In addition, they also appear to lengthen the life span of brain cells, possibly by increasing levels of nerve growth factor. In the past forty years, numerous studies have documented the ability of *Panax ginseng* to increase endurance and improve performance on a variety of physical and mental tasks, such as running, swimming, and performing mental arithmetic and logical deductions. When it was given to telegraph operators, they concentrated better, made fewer mistakes, and felt less fatigue. When students took it, they were able to focus their attention better and score higher on tests. Drivers stayed alert longer, and nurses adjusted more easily to night shifts.

These studies demonstrated that ginseng is most beneficial under conditions of stress, when the demand for adaptation is highest. A recent study conducted in Mexico suggests that ginseng improves both work performance and the overall quality of life. This double-blind study compared people taking multivitamin capsules to others taking multivitamins plus *Panax ginseng* extract. After four months, both groups showed improvements in quality of life, sense of well-being, mood, relationships, energy level, sexuality, and sleep, but the ginseng group experienced almost twice the benefit as those taking multivitamins alone.

Like its more famous cousin, Siberian ginseng (*Eleutherococcus senticosus*) has also been used in Asia for over 4,000 years for its tonic properties. Its active ingredients, called *eleutherosides,* function similarly to the ginsenosides in *Panax ginseng.* Siberian ginseng has been demonstrated to increase resistance to stress, fatigue, and disease. In clinical trials, subjects taking this herb have improved their ability to withstand stressors such as heat, noise, and motion. Other studies have shown increased mental alertness and work output, and improvements in the quality of work produced under stressful conditions.

The recommended dosage is 75 to 150 milligrams of *Panax ginseng* and/or 150 to 300 milligrams Siberian ginseng. Ginseng should be taken cyclically—daily for two months, then off for two weeks. This cycle may be repeated indefinitely. Siberian ginseng and *Panax ginseng* can be used alone or in combination with each other. They can also be used in combination with other herbs and nutrients, such as *Ginkgo biloba.*

High doses of ginseng may cause insomnia, elevated blood pressure, jitteriness, and heart palpitations. It should not be taken by people with hypertension, diabetes, or hypoglycemia without first consulting a doctor. If you are pregnant or nursing, consult a physician before using ginseng. Be aware that much of the ginseng on the market is derived from the lowest grade root that has been diluted, adulterated, or is totally void of active constituents. Make sure you choose a product containing an extract from the root that has been standardized for 7-percent ginsenosides in *Panax ginseng* or 0.8-percent eleutherosides in Siberian ginseng.

### St. John's Wort

Chronic stress often leads to depression or anxiety, and both of these conditions interfere with memory and mental function. In fact, it has been estimated that many cases of cognitive dysfunction and memory loss are misdiagnosed. In reality, they are caused by severe depression.

St. John's wort (*Hypericum perforatum*) is a safe, natural therapy that has been demonstrated to be an effective treatment for depression. It is as effective as prescription antidepressants, according to some studies. The *British Medical Journal* published a 1996 analysis of twenty-three clinical trials on St. John's wort, involving 1,757 patients. The trials demonstrated that the herb was three times as effective as a placebo in relieving the symptoms of depression. Even more important, in eight of these studies comparing St. John's wort to a prescription antidepressant, the herb was shown to be equally effective as the antidepressant—but with far fewer side effects and much less toxicity.

Like Prozac and other popular antidepressants, St. John's wort prolongs the activity of the neurotransmitter serotonin, which elevates mood. But it also appears to extend the actions of dopamine and norepinephrine, two other neurotransmitters that stimulate and energize the brain.

The recommended dosage of St. John's wort is 300 milligrams twice a day of an herbal extract standardized to contain 0.3-percent hypericin. If you are taking a prescription drug for depression, ask your doctor about St. John's wort before starting the herb. Also be aware that when taken in large doses for prolonged periods, this herb may cause sun sensitivity, especially in fair-skinned people.

### Kava

Kava (*Piper methysticum*) is nature's answer to tranquilizers and other medications used to treat anxiety. The roots of this plant, which is native to the South Pacific islands, contain unique phytochemicals called *kavalactones*. These work on the limbic system of the brain to produce a sense of calm and peacefulness. Unlike prescription anxiety drugs, which impair concentration and memory and have a host of other negative side effects, kava actually sharpens focus and improves memory. In a 1991 study, twenty-nine patients with symptoms of anxiety took 100 milligrams of kava three times a day, while twenty-nine others took a placebo. After four weeks, when compared to the placebo group, the patients taking kava had significant reductions in feelings of nervousness, heart palpitations, chest pains, dizziness, headaches, and gastrointestinal symptoms.

If you are suffering from anxiety, consider taking 150 milligrams of kava one to six times a day. Make sure you take an extract containing 30-percent kavalactones. Do not exceed two capsules in four hours or six capsules in twenty-four hours. Take kava for a maximum of three months, then discontinue for two to four weeks. This cycle may be repeated. It is important to avoid alcohol, barbiturates, psychiatric drugs, and other substances that affect the central nervous system when taking kava. Also, driving and operating heavy machinery is not recommended. For this reason, many people prefer to take kava in the evening.

## SUMMING IT UP

The natural biological response to stress is unavoidable. However, as this step of the program has shown, you can minimize the negative effects of chronic stress by using targeted supplements and practicing stress-reduction techniques. By normalizing stress hormone levels and taking the bite out of stress, not only will you protect your brain and sharpen your memory, but you will also notice improvements in mood and overall well-being.

Now let's move on to Step 8, where you'll discover another terrific stress reducer and brain booster—sleep.

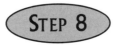

# Rejuvenate Your Brain
# With Sleep

*A s an intern and resident at busy teaching hospitals, I experienced
perhaps the most stressful years of my life. Like all doctors-in-train-
ing, I drew "night call" several times a week, which meant I got little or
no sleep every second or third night. Yet I was still required to keep up
with my studies, teaching duties, and patient care. Like the other interns
and residents, I got by. I looked upon this stage of medical training as the
way it was—good doctors simply rose to the occasion.*

Many studies have shown that sleep deprivation during medical training thwarts memory, impedes learning, clouds judgment, and places patients in jeopardy. In short, no one benefits
when physicians are routinely deprived of sleep. Foolhardy as
this practice may be, it is a deeply ingrained tradition—a trial by
fire and an initiation of young physicians into the fellowship of
medicine. And this sleep deprivation practice is unique to medicine. Imagine boarding a plane, knowing that an inexperienced
pilot-in-training who has just been forced to stay awake for twenty-four hours will be flying you from Chicago to Denver!

Inadequate sleep takes its toll on our bodies and our brains.
And interns and residents aren't the only ones who are sleep deprived. Lack of sleep is truly epidemic in this country, and we all
suffer the consequences. As you'll see in this step of the program,
quality sleep helps keep you mentally and physically sharp. First,
let's take a close look at what happens when we sleep.

## YOUR BRAIN NEVER SLEEPS

Before the 1930s, most scientists believed that sleep was a passive
condition. You went to bed tired and woke up rested. End of

story. So firm was the conviction that nothing happened during sleep that few scientists were even interested in studying it. In fact, before the 1950s, there was only one scientist, Nathaniel Kleitman, a professor of physiology at the University of Chicago, whose sole interest was the study of sleep. Dr. Kleitman, who established the world's first sleep laboratory, wrote of his discoveries in *Sleep and Wakefulness* in 1939. This book became the bible for sleep researchers everywhere. Today, Dr. Kleitman is considered the father of sleep research.

In 1953, a discovery was made in Dr. Kleitman's laboratory that revolutionized the field of sleep research. The discovery was *rapid eye movement sleep,* or *REM sleep,* which occurs for prolonged periods in infants and at regular intervals in the sleep of children and adults. Although the electroencephalograph (EEG), an instrument capable of detecting and recording minute changes in electrical activity in the brain, had been in use for approximately twenty years, until 1953 no one had bothered to conduct continuous EEG recordings during the night. To save paper and avoid having to stay up all night, readings were usually done only during the first hour of sleep, or for a few minutes every few hours. Consequently, the brain wave patterns characteristic of REM sleep had never been captured. That quickly changed, however, as researchers, intrigued by the phenomenon of rapid eye movements, honed in on the patterns of the night.

Hundreds of volunteers agreed to spend the night in sleep laboratories with tiny electrodes pasted to various parts of their head. What researchers found as they looked at the EEG readouts was astonishing. There was constant electrical activity throughout the night, even during the deepest sleep—and there were even periods of sleep that looked more like a state of heightened alertness than like sleep. Obviously something was going on in there.

## The Stages of Sleep

Researchers identified four different patterns of electrical activity that signified progressively deeper sleep. During Stages 1 and 2, called *short-wave sleep,* we make the transition from being awake to being in a light sleep. During these stages, EEG patterns show high-frequency brain waves that are extremely low (short) in amplitude (see Figure 4.3). In Stage 1, if asked to make a simple finger movement in response to a tone, we may succeed 50 percent of the time, but as we pass into Stage 2, we stop responding. Yet we can easily be roused from both Stage 1 and Stage 2 sleep, and may even deny that we were sleeping. Stages 3 and 4 are called *slow-wave sleep,* because they are characterized by low-frequency, high-amplitude (long) waves. In these deeper stages of sleep, responsiveness to the environment is minimal and it is difficult to be roused. A person awakened from Stage 4 sleep is likely to be groggy and disoriented.

Despite the wave changes that occur during Stages 1 through 4, they are often grouped together as *NREM sleep,* to differentiate them from the unique state of REM sleep. During REM sleep, your eyes make darting movements from side to side as if you are watching a movie inside your head. And in a sense, you are—you are dreaming. REM sleep is also called "paradoxical sleep" because the electrical activity that takes place during this stage is

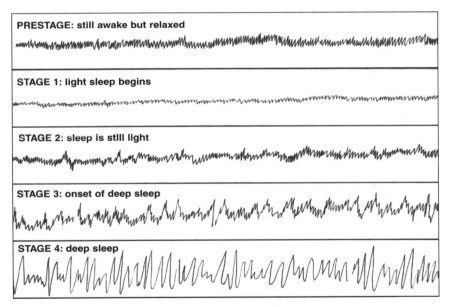

**Figure 4.3. Brain Waves and Stages of Sleep**
As seen in these simulated EEG printouts, each sleep stage has a distinctive brain-wave pattern. These stages recur in several cycles every night.

strikingly similar to a state of alertness and doesn't resemble sleep at all. Unlike deep sleep, in which your vital signs—heart rate, respiration rate, body temperature—are at their lowest, during REM sleep you are in a state of extreme arousal that resembles the "fight-or-flight" response described in Step 7. On the other hand, although you may move around during NREM sleep, your body is in a state of total muscular paralysis during REM sleep, as the motor cortex of your brain cuts off all nerve impulses to the spinal column. Your eyes are able to move only because the muscles that control them receive impulses from special nerve fibers that protrude from the brain stem.

Sleep cycles are roughly ninety minutes long and are repeated throughout the night. Each cycle starts with light sleep, then deepens until Stage 4 is reached. It then reverses direction, gradually becoming lighter until Stage 1 is reached. Each cycle ends with a dream. As the night goes on, the light stages shorten and the deep stages and REM sleep lengthen. We usually have our longest dream right before we wake up, and this is the one we are most likely to remember. Roughly 50 percent of our sleep time is spent in light sleep, 20 percent in deep sleep, and 30 percent in dreaming.

## The Chemistry of Sleep

Changes in brain wave patterns are not the only changes that occur while you sleep. There are also variations in the levels of certain neurotransmitters. For instance, levels of dopamine—the "energizing" neurotransmitter—decline, while levels of serotonin—the "happy" neurotransmitter—rise. Although the role of serotonin is more familiar as a mood regulator (both Prozac and St. John's wort target serotonin), this neurotransmitter is also vitally involved in regulating sleep. (Not surprisingly, one of the hallmarks of depression is insomnia.) Levels of acetylcholine, the neurotransmitter of learning and memory, rise during REM sleep and are likely the cause of the arousal pattern of brain waves that is so similar to our waking state.

Levels of certain hormones also change during the night. Perhaps the most dramatic changes occur in the hormone melatonin. The secretion of melatonin is keyed to light and darkness, and it plays a profound role in regulating the body's circadian rhythm—the twenty-four fluctuations in body temperature, hunger, energy, mood, and, of course, sleep and activity. In other words, the circadian rhythm is the body's "inner clock." Melatonin levels also seem to be choreographed by seasonal variations. When winter comes and the days grow shorter, our levels of melatonin are higher than they are in the summer. In fact, in some animals, the rise in melatonin levels ushers in winter hibernation, while spring, with its longer periods of daylight, has the opposite effect. Animals awaken from their slumber, the mating instinct kicks in, and they begin to reproduce.

Sleep also plays a role in regulating immunity. When you are sick, you tend to sleep more, which is the best thing you can do, because during sleep your immune system is at its most active. Studies of the effects of sleep deprivation on immune function have been conducted using laboratory animals, and the results are compelling. With only eight hours of sleep deprivation, the antibody response is weakened and remains this way for three days. Rats deprived of sleep invariably die by the twenty-first day, and the cause is usually an infection by a microorganism that the rat has successfully defeated many times before.

The same pattern holds true for humans. In a study of the effects of sleep deprivation on immunity, Dr. Zerrin Pelin, of the Sleep Disorders Unit at Istanbul University Medical School in Turkey, found that the percentage of natural killer cells—the "pit bulls" of the immune defense system—drops significantly after twenty-four hours of sleep deprivation. Even a modest loss of sleep, as little as five hours, results in a measurable reduction in natural immune responses. Epidemiological studies also bear this out.

Excluding variables such as age, alcohol use, and smoking, the people at greatest risk of dying are those who sleep the least. In one study conducted in Finland, 10,778 adults were followed for six years. Men who were poor sleepers were two and a half times more likely to die during this period than men who were good sleepers.

Women did not follow this trend in mortality, but for both

# Get Organized to Aid Memory

It is far easier to remember organized material than unorganized material. For example, learning the names of the United States is easier when done alphabetically than when done randomly, because the initial letters are a cue to the order.

The following shows how organizing material is helpful in remembering. Read the list of words in Box A at a steady rate, then read them a second time. Look away and write down as many words as you can remember in any order you like. Repeat the same process for the words in Box B.

### Box A—Unorganized Items

| beagle | Siamese | parakeet | pigeon | eagle |
| collie | poodle | Burmese | tiger | cockatoo |
| Maine coon | dove | cougar | cocker spaniel | parrot |
| German shepherd | canary | Persian | greyhound | |

### Box B—Organized Items

| DOG BREEDS | CAT BREEDS | BIRD BREEDS |
| --- | --- | --- |
| beagle | Burmese | canary |
| cocker spaniel | cougar | cockatoo |
| collie | Maine coon | dove |
| German shepherd | Persian | eagle |
| greyhound | Siamese | parakeet |
| poodle | tiger | parrot |

If you're like most people, you will find the organized entries in Box B easier to recall than the unstructured items in Box A. In addition to organizing the animals by breed, they have also been listed alphabetically to aid memory recall even further.

Organizational systems are useful for remembering lots of things. Use a family tree for remembering names of distant relatives, or organize items on a grocery list by separating them according to the different departments—produce, dairy, baked goods, etc.

sexes there was a definite correlation between poor sleep and poor health.

## POOR SLEEP EQUALS POOR COGNITIVE FUNCTION

British author Aldous Huxley observed, "That we are not much sicker and much madder than we are is due exclusively to that most blessed and blessing of all natural graces, sleep." Now that you understand the connection between sleep and physical health, let's look at the role sleep plays in your mental health. Why do you need sleep to keep your cognitive function sharp during the day? What happens when you don't get enough sleep?

While scientists have solid data on the negative effects of sleep deprivation on your memory and cognitive skills, they still haven't clarified precisely how and why sleep is so crucial to the brain. Clearly, the brain itself never sleeps. But it does wind down dramatically during slow-wave sleep, and researchers hypothesize that this is a restorative stage for the brain. If we are deprived of restful sleep one night, we tend to spend more time in deep, slow-wave sleep the next night. As we get older, the amount of time we spend in Stage 4 sleep steadily declines, and may completely disappear after age sixty. This may be one reason elderly people report more difficulty sleeping.

In contrast to slow-wave sleep, REM sleep seems to serve a different but equally important function. Volunteers who are persistently deprived of REM sleep become moody and depressed and may exhibit personality disorders, especially paranoia. While Freud saw dreams as meaningful symbols of the unconscious mind, others hypothesize that dreaming is a form of reverse learning. Accidental and meaningless neural connections made during the previous day are eliminated in order to maximize the efficiency of the thinking brain.

The effects of an occasional late night or early awakening on mood and cognition probably won't be noticeable—your brain is quite resilient. A good sleep the next night and you'll be feeling like yourself again. But many, if not most, of us are chronically sleep deprived, getting slightly less sleep than we need on a daily basis. And the effects of sleep deprivation are cumulative. If you're consistently getting an hour less sleep than you require, by the end of the week you will have lost the equivalent of one whole night's sleep. This is when sleep deprivation begins to take its toll. You'll feel more fatigued during the day, of course, but your mood will also suffer. You'll likely become more indecisive and less motivated. Most important, your cognitive ability and mental efficiency will be impaired.

At least fifty studies over the past decade have shown a consistent pattern: as the sleep debt increases, mental processes slow down, reaction time lengthens, and it becomes more difficult to focus attention on the task at hand. A wandering mind is likely to be a sleepy mind. Memory—especially working or short-term memory—is also impaired, and mental tasks that require remembering several pieces of information at a time become increasingly difficult. Creativity is also dampened, as sleep deprivation tends to put us on autopilot—we respond in preprogrammed ways rather than improvising on the spot. Any upset in the normal course of events is likely to cause a sort of brain "meltdown," as the mind simply cannot collect itself to deal with a novel situation. A sleep-deprived person is an accident waiting to happen, and statistics bear this out. As many as 100,000 motor vehicle accidents each year are attributed to sleepiness. And according to the National Sleep Foundation, more young people are killed every year by sleepy drivers than by drunk drivers.

## THE NATIONAL SLEEP DEBT

Most people keep a careful record of their budgetary credits and debits and take the time to balance their checkbook each month, rectifying any errors so that their account is up to date and they are not running a negative balance. Likewise, our federal budget is carefully scrutinized, and the deficits and occasional surpluses are prominently reported in our newspapers. But who's monitoring our national sleep debt? Certainly not the medical establishment.

Insomnia is largely ignored by doctors, as one review of medical records found. In one database of 10 million people who went to medical clinics, only seventy-three were diagnosed with sleep disorders. As Dr. William Denner of Stanford University, who conducted this review, observed, "In a population base this large, that's essentially zero." And yet surveys reveal that nearly one in three Americans sleep six hours or less per night during the work week—an hour and a half to two hours less than most people require.

According to another sleep researcher, Cornell University psychologist Dr. James Maas, almost every American is "short" one hour of sleep every night—a yearly debt of 365 hours, or more than two weeks of sleep lost every year.

## CAN LACK OF SLEEP MAKE YOU "DRUNK"?

Australian researchers have found a way to compare levels of fatigue with alcohol intoxication. It is hoped that this index will help predict the likelihood of workplace accidents. In this study, forty individuals underwent two experiments. In one, they were kept awake for twenty-eight hours; in the other, they consumed 10 to 15 grams of alcohol every thirty minutes until their average blood alcohol concentration reached 0.10 percent. Tests of hand-eye coordination were conducted at half-hour intervals throughout each experiment.

The researchers found that after ten hours of wakefulness, performance began to decline. At seventeen hours of wakefulness, the level of impairment was comparable to the deficit seen at a blood alcohol concentration of 0.05 percent, and at twenty-four hours, it was equivalent to a blood alcohol concentration of 0.10 percent—the level used by many states to define intoxication. As mentioned earlier in this chapter, the effects of sleep deprivation are cumulative, whether the lost sleep occurs during one night or is accumulated over a week. Those who are chronically running up a sleep debt are clearly suffering the effects in slower mental functioning.

## SLEEP MYTHS AND SLEEP FACTS

The rest of this chapter is devoted to solutions that will help you optimize your sleep for maximum performance during the day. But before I present these solutions, let me clear up a few of the most common myths surrounding sleep.

**Myth:** *Everyone needs eight hours of sleep each night.*
**Fact:** There is no ideal amount of sleep, although most adults need between four and nine hours. Whether you need six hours or eight hours of sleep to feel "normal," getting fewer hours than your body requires will affect your mental performance. There is also a great variation in the time of day we sleep. Some of us are "larks"—early to bed and early to rise—while others are "owls" who stay up late into the night and sleep late into the day. Ask a lark to stay up late, and you'll have to keep nudging him awake as the night goes on. Ask an owl to rise early, and you'll have one crabby owl. But virtually everyone sleeps some portion of the night. And there is a trend towards "larkdom" with age. Our body's circadian rhythm shifts slightly backward, so we go to sleep earlier and wake up earlier.

**Myth:** *Older adults need less sleep than younger adults.*
**Fact:** Infants need the greatest amount of sleep, and this need gradually declines until young adulthood. After that, the amount of sleep a given individual requires does not change significantly. Older adults don't need less sleep—they just have more difficulty sleeping. Chronic pain, certain medications, and declines in levels of hormones and neurotransmitters contribute to poor sleep in the elderly. As the body's circadian rhythm shifts backward, it also flattens out, with less dramatic peaks and valleys. Consequently, older adults tend to wake more easily and more often than young or middle-aged adults.

**Myth:** *After a while, your body adjusts to shift work.*
**Fact:** The body has a natural wake/sleep cycle that is timed with changes in light and temperature. In essence, we are programmed to sleep at night. Studies have concluded that people who work night shifts perform less efficiently than day workers. These workers are required to sleep during the time of day when the body and brain are most primed for activity.

**Myth:** *Younger people are not as affected by poor sleep as older people.*
**Fact:** Actually, the opposite is true. Numerous studies have demonstrated that, while on the average, older people score lower on tests of memory and cognitive function than younger adults, their scores after sleep deprivation or sleep interruption do not drop as significantly as those of younger adults. In addition, younger adults tend to overestimate their ability to perform while sleep deprived.

**Myth:** *Cramming the night before a test or a presentation is the best way to remember things the next day.*
**Fact:** "Burning the midnight oil" to cram facts into your brain is less likely to improve memory than a good night's sleep. Studies have shown that sleep deprivation immediately after learning results in inferior performance. While you can't learn while sleeping, you can promote the processing, consolidation, and storage of memories. Review the most important moments of your day just before sleeping, and let your subconscious brain do the rest.

## HOW TO GET A GOOD NIGHT'S SLEEP

Now that we've cleared up some common myths about sleep, let's look at the most common sleep disturbers. Then I'll give you some tips you can implement to ensure a good night's sleep.

### Eliminate Sleep Disrupters

The coffee in your pantry, the beer in your refrigerator, and the medication on your nightstand are just three of the bandits that steal your sleep away. As mentioned earlier, caffeine is a stimulant that may offer a short-term benefit but quickly becomes a detriment to cognition and memory. Caffeine enters your bloodstream immediately, produces a noticeable effect in thirty minutes, and remains in the bloodstream for six hours. Many people who are chronically sleep deprived rely on a "jolt of java" to keep themselves awake during the day. Chances are, if you need caffeine to keep you going throughout the day, you're not getting

enough sleep at night. I highly recommend that you give up caffeine or limit yourself to a maximum of one cup of coffee (or, better yet, green tea) in the morning, and switch to herbal teas and
water for the remainder of the day. Keep in mind that there is also
caffeine in black and green teas, most sodas, chocolate, and some
over-the-counter and prescription medicines.

Nicotine is another stimulant that impairs nighttime sleep
and daytime cognitive performance. Obviously, it's not possible
to smoke and sleep at the same time, so levels of nicotine drop
during the night, leading to withdrawal symptoms. In a survey
conducted by researchers at the University of Kentucky, 869 individuals aged fourteen to eighty-four were queried about their
health, sleep habits, and daytime function. Cigarette smokers
were significantly more likely than nonsmokers to report difficulty in falling sleep, difficulty staying asleep, daytime sleepiness, minor accidents, and depression. To all the other excellent
reasons for kicking the habit—reducing your risk of cancer, heart
disease, and emphysema, and improving your senses of smell
and taste—add this one. If you are a smoker, you simply must
decide to quit.

A glass of wine before bed may help you fall asleep, but any
more than that disrupts sleep significantly. Alcohol primarily
suppresses REM sleep. In addition, alcohol increases the risk of
restless leg syndrome, a condition in which periodic leg movements occur frequently during sleep. In one study, women who
had two or more alcoholic drinks per night were three times as
likely to have twenty or more periodic leg movements per hour
than women who did not. People who have restless leg syndrome are generally poor sleepers.

Besides what you put in your body, what you put in your
bedroom may prevent you from getting a good night's sleep.
Take that television at the foot of the bed, which some people
insist helps them fall asleep. The truth is, light of any kind—
whether it's coming from the television, the lamp on your nightstand, or the streetlight outside your window—lowers levels of
melatonin, the hormone that regulates sleep. Turn the television
off, make sure the shades are drawn when you go to bed, and if
there are sources of light you can't block out, consider wearing an

eye mask. There's also a psychological reason for why you shouldn't watch television in bed. Your mind is extremely susceptible to the power of suggestion. If you eat, watch television, or read in bed, the association in your mind between your bed and sleep will be weakened by activities associated with wakefulness. Don't get into bed until you're ready to sleep, and your brain will be primed for the restful night to come.

Now let's look at some safe, natural remedies for insomnia that will help you maintain your mental edge and a sharp memory.

## Exercise to Sleep Better

Vigorous aerobic exercise is perhaps the single most powerful and effective antidote for insomnia. As you saw in Step 7, high levels of stress impair sleep. The reverse is also true—impaired sleep increases stress levels. Physical exercise is a healthy and efficient way to alleviate stress and address two other common sleep stealers, depression and anxiety. The evidence that aerobic exercise aids sleep is strong. In one study conducted by Stanford University researchers, forty-three people, aged fifty to seventy-six, who commonly experienced sleep disturbances, were divided into an exercise group and a sedentary group. Exercisers did thirty to forty minutes of low-impact aerobics four times a week, while the other group remained sedentary. After sixteen weeks, those in the exercise group reported measurable improvements in sleep. The time it took the exercisers to fall asleep fell from twenty-eight minutes to less than fifteen minutes.

To get the benefits of exercise, you need to get your heart pumping and your blood flowing. Find a place to fit it into your schedule that works best for you, but don't exercise during the last two hours before you go to bed, as this may make falling asleep more difficult.

## Increase Serotonin Levels

As mentioned before, serotonin is the "happy" neurotransmitter, and low levels of this chemical messenger are associated with

## Insomnia and Prescription Drugs

The most common prescription drugs used to treat insomnia are barbiturates (sedatives) and benzodiazepines (tranquilizers). While these drugs may promote sleep in the short term, they actually disrupt sleep cycles and impair daytime functioning over the long run. Like alcohol, barbiturates suppress REM sleep. Benzodiazepines have a more profound effect on slow-wave sleep, although they also affect REM sleep. Most of these drugs can cause rebound insomnia, especially during the last third of the night, when both slow-wave sleep and REM sleep are at their peak.

Besides their counterproductive effects on sleep, prescription sedatives and tranquilizers significantly impair cognitive function during the day. Common side effects of barbiturates include drowsiness, dizziness, lethargy, headache, vertigo, severe depression, anxiety, irritability, and mental impairment. Elderly patients are at greater risk of these and other side effects, such as confusion and excitation.

Benzodiazepines are prescribed to almost one in five adults over age sixty-five. These drugs are extremely addictive and cause withdrawal symptoms after as little as one week of use. Even if taken for a short time, they can cause daytime drowsiness, fatigue, loss of muscular coordination, and impaired cognition and memory. Almost 14 percent of all hip fractures and 16,000 automobile accidents per year are linked to these and other prescription drugs that affect the mind.

depression. People who are depressed often have insomnia, and antidepressants known as *selective serotonin reuptake inhibitors (SSRIs)*, such as Prozac, Paxil, and Zoloft, tend to promote sleep. Independent of its role in mood, serotonin plays a key role in regulating sleep.

Serotonin is derived from the amino acid tryptophan. As blood levels of this amino acid rise, there is a corresponding elevation in levels of serotonin, prompting sleep. Supplemental tryptophan used to be a popular over-the-counter sleep aid.

However, in 1990, the Food and Drug Administration banned this amino acid when one Japanese company produced batches of it that were contaminated with a toxic element (tryptophan itself is completely safe). Tryptophan is now available through compounding pharmacies, but it requires a prescription, which may be difficult to obtain from a conventional physician.

Another readily available way to increase serotonin levels and promote sleep is to supplement with 5-hydroxytryptophan (5-HTP). The conversion of tryptophan to serotonin actually occurs in two steps. First, tryptophan is converted to 5-HTP, then 5-HTP is converted to serotonin. Studies have reached conflicting conclusions about which of these two compounds is more effective in promoting sleep. Because 5-HTP is extremely safe and widely available, I recommend trying it first. Look for natural 5-HTP, which is derived from the seeds of *Griffonia simplicifolia*, a West African plant.

Ten times as strong as tryptophan, 5-HTP requires a relatively small dosage to encourage sleep. I recommend starting with 50 milligrams at bedtime. If needed, gradually work up to a maximum dose of 100 milligrams. Although higher doses are sometimes taken throughout the day to ease depression, this should be sufficient to facilitate sleep. If you are taking a prescription antidepressant, do not take tryptophan or 5-HTP without consulting your physician. Vitamins $B_5$ and $B_6$ are also involved in the synthesis of serotonin, so be sure to take a multivitamin that contains these vitamins, as well.

## Reset Your Body Clock With Melatonin

In Eastern traditions, the pineal gland, a tiny structure embedded in the center of the brain, is known as "the third eye"—an accurate description of a gland that responds to changes in light. When darkness falls, the pineal gland boosts its secretion of the hormone melatonin. Levels of melatonin peak between the hours of 1 AM and 5 AM, then gradually fall as the sun rises. As with other hormones, melatonin production declines dramatically with age. At the age of forty, the body produces approximately one-sixth the melatonin it did during the teen years. Levels continue to decline into old age, which may be one reason why sleep problems are so common among the elderly.

A number of studies have shown that supplemental melatonin decreases the time required to fall asleep and produces a deep and restful sleep without the side effects of prescription sedatives. Because melatonin regulates circadian rhythms, it is especially useful for shift workers and travelers suffering from jet lag. One study, published in the *British Medical Journal,* examined the effects of melatonin on seventeen travelers flying from San Francisco to London. Eight subjects took 5 milligrams of melatonin at 6:00 PM, California time, for three days prior to departure. For three days upon their arrival in London, they took the same dose between the hours of 10:00 PM and midnight, England time. Nine subjects were given a placebo, with the same instructions. At the conclusion of the study, six of the nine subjects taking a placebo rated their jet lag as above 50 on a scale of 1 to 100 (with 100 being the most severe). In contrast, none of the eight subjects on melatonin rated their jet lag as higher than 17.

Melatonin is also a potent antioxidant. It boosts immune function and counters the harmful effects of stress—another way in which it protects your brain and cognitive function. The average recommended melatonin dose is 3 milligrams, but I suggest that you start at a lower dose of 0.5 milligrams, and increase dosage (if necessary) to no more than 6 milligrams. Melatonin should be taken thirty to sixty minutes before going to sleep.

Never take melatonin during the day unless you do work at night, then take it thirty to sixty minutes before your usual bedtime. If you are traveling across time zones, take melatonin thirty to sixty minutes before going to sleep for the first three days in the new time zone. I don't recommend melatonin for those under age forty, or for anyone who suffers from mental illness, severe allergies, autoimmune diseases, lymphoma, or leukemia. Women who are pregnant or nursing, and those taking prescription steroid drugs should avoid melatonin.

## Consider Nature's Sleeping Pills

There are a number of natural agents that facilitate sleep. One is valerian. It is the most widely used sleep aid in Europe, and for good reason. Valerian contains a powerful sleep-inducing compound called valeric acid, which is capable of binding to the same receptor sites in the brain as benzodiazepine drugs, such as Valium. (The similarity between their names is no accident!) Yet unlike benzodiazepines, valerian does not produce the impaired mental function, morning hangover, and dependency that are characteristic of these prescription drugs.

Valerian's effectiveness has been verified in numerous studies. In one study that included sixty individuals with insomnia, twenty received a combination of valerian root (160 milligrams) and lemon balm (80 milligrams); twenty received a benzodiazepine drug, and twenty received a placebo. The valerian combination was as effective as the drug, and it also increased sleep Stages 3 and 4—the deepest stages. However, the herbal preparation did not produce daytime sleepiness or impair concentration or physical performance.

The recommend dose of valerian is 130 to 150 milligrams of an extract that has been standardized to contain 0.8-percent valeric acid. Valerian is safe and has no known side effects. It is best taken thirty to forty-five minutes before going to bed.

Another natural agent that facilitates sleep is magnesium, which relaxes muscles and is especially effective at preventing and alleviating restless leg syndrome. The recommended dose, as described in Step 2, is 500 milligrams per day.

Other herbal sleep enhancers include kava, chamomile, hops, and passionflower. A nice, relaxing cup of one of these herbal teas thirty to sixty minutes before going to bed melts away stress and prepares you for a peaceful sleep.

## SUMMING IT UP

As this step has shown, it is very important not to underestimate the role of sleep in mental function. It's one factor that busy people tend to discount. Keep in mind that a good night's sleep makes all the difference in the world in your mental outlook and cognitive function.

## STEP 9

# Enhance Brain Function With Hormones

*When Betty went through menopause, she "fell apart." This healthy, composed woman became a bundle of nerves and emotions. She had repeated hot flashes during the day and disrupted sleep at night. She was testy and impatient with her family and less productive at work—she just couldn't seem to concentrate. After six months of suffering in silence, she came to my clinic and was started on natural estrogen and progesterone replacement therapy. Her symptoms completely disappeared, and her mental clarity and focus returned.*

*Hugh was in his early fifties when he started to slow down. He felt tired, lethargic, and unfocused. An avid cyclist, he was getting nowhere in his training in spite of stepping up his workouts. Given his age and the fact that his blood level of testosterone was low, he was encouraged to consider a trial of testosterone replacement. Hugh returned to the clinic a few months later with renewed energy, drive, and focus. Mentally and physically, he felt like an eighteen-year-old again.*

Chapter 2 presented the four primary processes that are involved in the aging and degeneration of our bodies—oxidation, methylation defects, inflammation, and glycation. In subsequent chapters, you saw how you can control or at least slow down these processes and protect your body and brain from the ravages of aging. This step of the program addresses another important factor in the aging process—the decline in the body's production of hormones.

Hormones are chemicals produced by the glands of the endocrine system. Secreted into the bloodstream in minute amounts and carried to receptor sites in various areas of the body, hormones affect virtually every system in the body, including the brain and central nervous system. Drops in hormone levels are one of the most predictable indicators of aging and the basis for yet another explanation of aging—the biological clock theory, also known as programmed senescence.

According to this theory, hormones control the entire process, from birth to death. Growth hormone is produced in abundance during the rapid growth stages of childhood and adolescence. It falls off around age twenty, when the body stops growing. Estrogen and progesterone levels rise as a girl enters puberty, remain steady during her reproductive years, and then decline as she reaches her forties or fifties. Testosterone is another hormone that gears up in males during adolescence and begins a gradual decline after the mid-twenties. DHEA, pregnenolone, and thyroid follow a similar curve in both men and women. All of these hormonal ebbs and flows are orchestrated by the hormone melatonin, which is produced in the pineal gland. Melatonin signals and cues the production of other hormones.

This theory is pretty tidy in many respects, and whether or not it truly explains the aging process is immaterial. What is important is that the signs and symptoms of aging accelerate once hormone levels fall off. Bones become brittle, hearts get weaker, muscles atrophy, sex drive and function plummet, and memory loss and cognitive deficits dramatically increase.

Hormone replacement therapy is powerful medicine. Unfortunately, with the exception of thyroid, and estrogen and progesterone for postmenopausal women, hormone therapy is completely ignored by conventional physicians. Men are only rarely offered testosterone, while hormones like DHEA and pregnenolone are vilified. As a result of this bias, patients are missing out on an entire category of therapeutic agents that have the potential of making a true difference in their health. I use a wide variety of hormones in my medical practice to address a diverse range of medical conditions. Thousands of my patients over the age of forty-five, both men and women, have benefited tremendously from hormone therapy. This step of the program takes a look at the hormones most intimately involved in brain function (see Figure 4.4) and shows how supplementing with safe, natural forms of these hormones can dramatically benefit your memory and mental function.

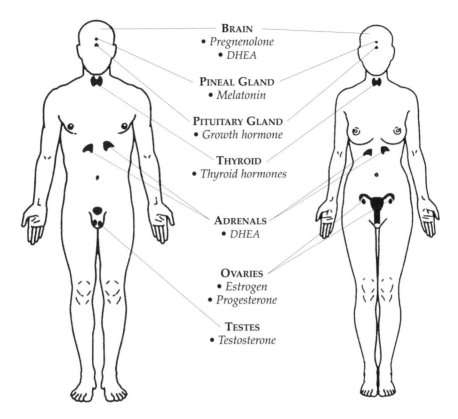

**Figure 4.4. Endocrine Glands and the Hormones They Secrete**

## PREGNENOLONE—THE MEMORY HORMONE

Possibly the most powerful memory-enhancing hormone of all, pregnenolone is a steroid hormone, synthesized in the adrenal glands from cholesterol. It is considered a precursor hormone because from it, DHEA, estrogen, testosterone, and other hormones are made, as illustrated in Figure 4.5. When the body's production of pregnenolone lags, as it inevitably does with age, production of these other hormones declines as well.

Unlike most of the other steroid hormones, pregnenolone, which is sometimes called a *neurosteroid,* is also produced in the brain and spinal cord. This tells us something right away about its importance to the brain. One way in which pregnenolone affects cognitive function is through its actions on the brain's

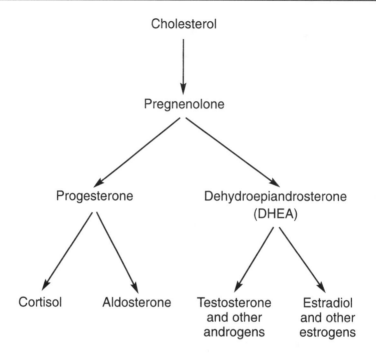

**Figure 4.5. The Hormonal Cascade**

As this figure shows, all steroid hormones are made from pregnenolone.

chemical messengers and their receptor sites. In a number of animal studies, pregnenolone was shown to enhance the release of the neurotransmitter acetylcholine, which is involved in learning and memory.

Pregnenolone also affects GABA, an inhibitory neurotransmitter that calms down activity in the brain, as well as aspartate, an excitatory neurotransmitter that stimulates it. Thus, pregnenolone has a stabilizing, balancing effect on the brain as it occupies both aspartate and GABA receptor sites. Pregnenolone also has protective effects on nerve cells, and it is being explored as a treatment for spinal cord injuries. Rather astounding animal studies have demonstrated that, in combination with drugs, pregnenolone suppresses the inflammation associated with such injuries, and injured animals have been restored to near-normal function.

Eugene Roberts, Ph.D., at the City of Hope Hospital in Duarte,

California, has been involved in pregnenolone research for years and has found it to be the most potent hormone for memory enhancement. In a 1992 study, Dr. Roberts and colleagues gave mice supplemental pregnenolone, DHEA, progesterone, estrogen, or testosterone and then had them run through a maze. All of these hormones improved memory and maze performance in the laboratory animals, but none of them improved the animals' memory as well as the pregnenolone.

Human studies also give pregnenolone a thumbs-up. One of the earliest experiments on pregnenolone and memory was conducted using a flight simulator. Study subjects included both pilots and people with no flight experience, who were required to track a moving target by manipulating a joystick—much like the ones used in the video games our children and grandchildren play. Their performance was scored on the percentage of time they stayed with the randomly moving target over the period of an hour. If you've ever tried such a video game, you know that this requires intense concentration and quick reflexes, and it's quite tiring. It taxes concentration and hand-eye coordination.

The study ran in three phases over two and a half months. The subjects were tested while on a placebo during the first phase, 50 milligrams of daily pregnenolone during the second phase, and back on the placebo during the final phase. During the first phase, they stayed on target an average of 25 to 35 percent. While taking pregnenolone during the second phase, the scores jumped to 35 to 50 percent. During the second placebo phase, the scores stayed at the higher level for several days before falling back down to the baseline. This suggests that the effects of pregnenolone are sustained for a time after you stop taking it. An interesting aside is that the pilots in the study reported that while they were taking pregnenolone, they found that their real-life flying skills were sharper, and they felt less fatigue while on the job.

More recently, researchers at St. Louis University demonstrated that pregnenolone also improves memory and concentration in people over age fifty. Women performed better on tests of verbal recall after taking this supplement, while men's scores in spatial tasks improved.

If you are experiencing memory loss or feel you are losing your mental edge, I recommend that you consider trying pregnenolone, starting at a dose of 20 milligrams per day. If no improvement is noted after two months, gradually increase the dosage to 50 milligrams. Although pregnenolone is quite safe—study subjects administered 500 milligrams per day had no adverse effects—I advise staying in the 50-milligram range. I do not recommend pregnenolone or any of the steroid hormones discussed in this chapter for most people who are younger than forty-five, as their own bodies produce adequate amounts of hormones.

## DHEA—THE REJUVENATOR

Another powerful memory-enhancing hormone is DHEA (dehydroepiandrosterone). It is not to be confused with DHA, the important brain fat that was discussed in Step 4. DHEA is a steroid hormone that is produced in the adrenal glands, but is also synthesized in the skin and the brain. It is the second rung of the "hormonal cascade," as seen in Figure 4.5. Pregnenolone is converted into DHEA, which, in turn, may be converted into estrogen and testosterone.

DHEA is produced in far greater abundance than any of the other adrenal hormones, yet for years its functions were unknown. It was believed to be only a storehouse from which the body could produce other hormones, rather than having functions of its own. Recent research, however, has pinpointed DHEA as an extremely powerful hormone in its own right. It counteracts the detrimental effects of stress and boosts immunity. Low levels of DHEA are associated with a variety of medical conditions, including cardiovascular disease, obesity, diabetes, lipid disorders, immune dysfunction, autoimmune disorders, osteoporosis, and cancer.

Patients with Alzheimer's disease also often have low DHEA levels, as the following study, performed by researchers at the National Institutes of Mental Health in Bethesda, Maryland, illustrates. First, the researchers determined the blood levels of DHEA sulfate (the most common measurement of this hormone) in ten patients with Alzheimer's disease. They then compared them to the levels of ten healthy people of the same age and sex, and nine young healthy people. As expected, the younger group's DHEA sulfate levels were more than twice as high as either of the older group's. But more significantly, the DHEA levels of the individuals with Alzheimer's disease were an average of 48-percent lower than those of healthy people the same age. Studies are now looking at whether DHEA levels affect the course of Alzheimer's disease. They are also examining supplemental DHEA as a therapy for Alzheimer's and other less severe forms of memory loss.

Exactly how DHEA affects your brain is also under investigation. We do know that it counters the harmful chemicals that chronic stress unleashes. As described earlier, stress hormones have particularly damaging effects on the hippocampus—the area of the brain that processes memory—and DHEA appears to protect this important structure. Test-tube studies also show that when brain cells are exposed to DHEA, the growth of new axons and dendrites is stimulated.

Supplemental DHEA has been shown to increase learning and memory in laboratory animals and help older mice navigate mazes as well as younger mice. Although human studies are limited, supplemental DHEA has also been shown to have a positive effect on memory in older people. In one small study of patients with memory loss and depression carried out at the University of California at San Francisco, patients taking 30 to 90 milligrams of DHEA daily for four weeks experienced dramatic improvements in mood and memory.

I recommend DHEA extensively in my medical practice, and the most common remark I hear from my patients is that it just makes them feel better—more alert and clearheaded. The usual starting dose of DHEA is 25 to 50 milligrams a day for women and 50 to 100 milligrams a day for men, although some patients notice benefits with as little as 10 milligrams. Purported "DHEA precursors" from Mexican yam and other sources have little to no effect on DHEA blood levels. If you're going to take DHEA, make sure it's pure pharmaceutical grade. I test my patients' blood levels at the onset of treatment and again in three months to make sure they are taking the proper dose. We try to maintain blood levels at the high-normal range for a young adult, regardless of age.

DHEA has received some bad press in the past few years, and its safety has been questioned. However, all the medical literature indicates that it is quite safe, even at doses much higher than those I recommend. Larger doses may have temporary masculin-izing effects in women, such as growth of facial hair or skin breakouts. This is because, as Figure 4.5 illustrates, DHEA cas-cades into other hormones, including testosterone. Although there is no evidence that DHEA contributes to cancer, it is con-verted into testosterone, so I advise men with prostate cancer to avoid it. In addition, most people under age forty-five are pro-ducing adequate levels of the hormone and don't need supple-mentation.

## ESTROGEN AND PROGESTERONE: WOMEN'S GUARDIAN ANGELS

Not too many years ago, estrogen and progesterone were consid-ered to be involved strictly in female reproduction and sexual characteristics. We now know that these hormones play im-portant roles in bone remodeling, cardiovascular health, and brain function. Let's look at estrogen first, as dozens of recent studies have clarified its remarkable effects on the brain.

Estrogen protects brain cells from free-radical activity, and it enhances production of acetylcholine. This hormone also in-creases the production of nerve growth factor, which nurtures and protects neurons. Researchers at the National Institutes of Health recently discovered that estrogen actually stimulates dendrite branching in the hippocampus, the area of the brain associated with memory and the first to be affected by Alz-heimer's disease.

It is clear that estrogen replacement therapy improves cogni-tive function in postmenopausal women. A 1997 study looked at the effects of supplemental estrogen on 116 women over age forty, compared to 172 nonusers of the same age. Every six years from 1978 to 1991, these women were given memory tests. They were asked to look at ten different shapes for a few seconds, then draw them on a piece of paper. Scores for all women declined with age, as expected, but the women who took estrogen scored better on this test of visual memory—and they continued to do so over time.

Another study demonstrated that estrogen also helps preserve language and abstract reasoning. Dr. Diane M. Jacobs authored a study published in the February 1998 issue of *Neurology*, which involved 727 postmenopausal women who had no significant memory problems. Some of the women were on estrogen replacement; some were not. They were given tests to measure their language, memory, and abstract reasoning skills at the study's onset and then again two and a half years later. Researchers found that the women taking estrogen scored consistently higher on these tests. They concluded that estrogen therapy might help postmenopausal women maintain memory and cognitive function.

The relationship between estrogen replacement and Alzheimer's disease has also been explored. Scientists from the University of Southern California School of Medicine have followed 8,877 female members of a retirement community since 1981. In one of their studies, they focused on the 2,529 women who had died as of 1992, and found that 138 of them had had Alzheimer's disease or some form of dementia. The researchers then determined which women had taken supplemental estrogen and found that those who had been on estrogen replacement had a 30-percent decrease in the incidence of dementia. A more recent study, conducted as part of the Baltimore Longitudinal Study on Aging (discussed in Chapter 1) pegged the protection offered by estrogen replacement to be even greater, as high as 46 percent.

Most of the existing studies on estrogen's effects on Alzheimer's disease have examined its role in protection against Alzheimer's disease, rather than as treatment for existing disease. However, promising research is now exploring the possibility that estrogen both repairs and protects neurons. Because it improves cerebral blood flow, elevates nerve growth factor, supports neuronal function and growth, protects nerve cells against injury, and stimulates the transport of glucose in the brain, estrogen has a bright future as a therapy for Alzheimer's disease and other forms of dementia.

The other feminine hormone, progesterone, and its role in cognitive function have not been studied to the degree that estrogen has. However, it is known that receptor sites for this hormone do exist in the brain. It is also produced in the central nervous system and is involved in its communication network. Furthermore, progesterone stimulates the formation of the nerve's protective myelin sheaths. Perhaps most important, estrogen should always be taken with progesterone. The cardinal rule of hormone replacement therapy is to try to mimic nature as closely as possible. Since both hormones are produced in a woman's body, they should both be supplemented. They keep each other in balance, and progesterone protects against the stimulating effects estrogen has on the uterine lining when taken alone.

I recommend that postmenopausal women and women who have had hysterectomies seriously consider the benefits of estrogen and progesterone replacement therapy. Generally, the onset of menopause is around age fifty, and a woman can expect to live at least twenty-five more years in a state of hormone deficiency. I am extremely cautious about the types of hormone replacement my patients use. I prescribe only natural hormones, which are identical to the molecular structure of the hormones produced by the human body. I believe the top-selling hormone drugs, such as Premarin (derived from the urine of pregnant horses) and Provera (a synthetic progestin used to replace progesterone), do not belong in a woman's body. I offer my patients a combination of 80-percent estriol, a safe, weak form of estrogen, and 20-percent estradiol, a more potent estrogen. Estrogen should always be balanced with progesterone, so, along with this, I add natural progesterone.

Most physicians are unfamiliar with natural hormones, so you might have to look for a doctor experienced with these hormones and a compounding pharmacy to make them up. Natural estrogen and progesterone are far safer than the pharmaceuticals and equally effective. Although estrogen and oral progesterone are available by prescription only, natural progesterone creams that are rubbed into the skin are sold in health food stores.

## TESTOSTERONE—MEN'S PROTECTOR

Testosterone is the hormone that gives men "masculine" characteristics, such as whiskers, muscles, deep voices, strong sex drives, and streaks of aggression. As testosterone levels decline with age, men lose muscle mass, their libidos shift into low gear, and they experience decreases in energy and motivation. This is a condition known as *andropause*.

Andropause is essentially the male equivalent of menopause, and although few men will admit to it (and many conventional physicians deny its existence), my twenty-five years of working with older male patients have convinced me that andropause is every bit as real as menopause. It even has some of the same symptoms as menopause, including fatigue, depression, irritability, lack of focus and drive, and aches and pains. Reduced sexual interest, enjoyment, and performance are also common. Furthermore, after andropause, the incidence of heart disease, osteoporosis, and Alzheimer's and other degenerative diseases increases. This is due, at least in part, to low testosterone levels.

Research on testosterone's activity in the brain is still in its infancy. We do know that this hormone occupies specific receptor sites in the male brain. And according to William Regelson, M.D., in his excellent book, *The Superhormone Promise*, recent studies suggest that the presence of testosterone in the brain may explain at least one of the differences between the way in which men and women think. It has long been recognized that males are generally better than females at visual spatial tasks, things that involve orienting objects, and seeing things in three dimensions. Generally speaking, young boys are adept at tossing balls at targets and building Lego figures from pictures. Older boys excel in reading maps and throwing darts. As testosterone levels decline with age, men consistently do worse on tests of spatial ability. However, their performance is bolstered on such tests when they are given supplemental testosterone. Other studies suggest that supplemental testosterone may also improve verbal recall in men and protect against Alzheimer's disease.

Two areas in which supplemental testosterone is clearly beneficial are mood and energy levels. Studies submitted to the FDA for approval of the Androderm testosterone patch showed marked improvement in these two areas. After twelve months of use, depression scores were cut almost in half while reported fatigue fell from 79 to 10 percent.

If you are a man over the age of forty-five, I suggest that you have your testosterone level evaluated. If it is below the level of a young adult, regardless of your age, consider a trial of supplemental testosterone. For my patients, I prescribe only natural testosterone, which comes in lozenges, sprays, gels, and patches. The lozenges, which most of my patients prefer, are tucked into the mouth between the gums and cheek. The testosterone is then absorbed through the mucosa of the cheek into the bloodstream. It bypasses the gastrointestinal tract, eliminating the possibility of liver toxicity. The gels, sprays, and patches are applied to the skin. I do not recommend oral testosterone, which can be toxic to the liver, or testosterone injections, which may be converted to less than desirable compounds in the body.

## THYROID HORMONES—THE ENERGIZERS

The first hormones you should have checked if you are having problems with your memory are thyroid hormones. These hormones play multiple roles, but they are primarily involved in metabolism and the rate of chemical changes in the body. Hyperthyroidism, caused by an overproduction of thyroid hormones, speeds things up—your heartbeat, the rate at which your body burns food for energy, and your overall metabolism. This is a serious but relatively rare condition. Much more common is hypothyroidism, the result of inadequate secretion of thyroid hormones. Low levels of these important hormones cause a slowing down of your system and result in fatigue, depression, slow heartbeat, intolerance to cold, weight gain, hair loss, constipation, difficulty in concentrating, and memory loss.

Hypothyroidism affects men and women of all ages, but it is most common in older women. It is a significant factor in loss of cognitive function in the elderly, yet it is often overlooked. While every doctor will pick up dramatically low thyroid levels on laboratory exams, many miss the clinical signs of hypothyroidism when lab values are in the low-to-normal range. I believe that even if lab tests are within low normal limits, patients with signs and symptoms of low thyroid, which include memory and concentration deficits, should be given a trial of thyroid replacement.

The most common type of thyroid supplementation is Synthroid (levothyroxine), a synthetic version of T4, which is a single thyroid hormone. I would never recommend Synthroid for my patients. Instead, I prescribe Armor Thyroid (Forest Pharmaceuticals), a natural thyroid preparation made from porcine thyroid that contains the full gamut of thyroid hormones. Supporters of the synthetics argue that T4 is the most active thyroid hormone. True, but it's not the only thyroid hormone, and the clinical response to natural thyroid often stands head and shoulders above the synthetic type. Getting your doctor to recommend thyroid supplementation—and especially natural thyroid—when blood levels are in the low-to-normal range may be a challenge. However, in many cases, a clinical trial of low-dose natural thyroid may boost metabolism enough to improve memory and get back your mental edge.

An easy way to determine your thyroid function, and one you can do at home, is to measure your basal body temperature. This method was developed by Dr. Broda Barnes, a pioneer in endocrine research. Here's what to do. Before you go to bed at night, shake down a regular oral thermometer (or for easier reading, purchase a basal thermometer) and leave it within easy reach of your bed. Immediately upon awakening in the morning—before getting out of bed or even stretching—place the thermometer under your armpit for ten minutes. Do this for three to five consecutive days. (Menstruating women should do this during the first four days of their periods for greatest reliability.) Record your daily temperatures and average them. Normal is 97.8°F to 98.2°F. If your average temperature is less than 97.8°F, you may be hypothyroid and might benefit from supplemental thyroid. For more information on natural thyroid, contact the Broda O. Barnes, MD, Research Foundation, Inc., PO Box 98, Trumbull, CT 06611; 203–261–2101.

## HOW TO OBTAIN NATURAL HORMONES

Some hormones, such as pregnenolone, DHEA, natural progesterone cream, and melatonin, discussed in Step 8, may be purchased over the counter in your drugstore or health food store. The others, including estrogen, oral progesterone, testosterone, and thyroid hormones, require a prescription. Hormone replacement therapy is one area in which the conventional and the alternative in medicine collide. As I stated before, most conventional physicians are resistant to the idea of prescribing any type of hormone other than estrogen, progesterone, and thyroid. On the other hand, many doctors who practice alternative medicine find the broader use of hormone replacement therapy invaluable in the treatment of patients over the age of forty-five, when production of these rejuvenating compounds begins to decline. I don't advocate super-dosing; I want only to return my patients' hormone levels to those of a young adult. If you are unable to work with your doctor in this matter, I suggest you look for a physician who is experienced in natural hormone replacement.

There is another area in which those who practice alternative and conventional treatments disagree. Conventional physicians routinely recommend pharmaceutical synthetic hormones. As an advocate of alternative medicine, I believe in replacing hormones in forms that are as close to those your body produces as possible. Natural, human-identical hormones work as well, if not better than, the synthetic types, but they are much safer and cause far fewer unwanted side effects. Natural hormones are available from compounding pharmacists, who prepare individual orders per the physician's prescription. For organizations that can direct you to both physicians trained in natural therapies and compounding pharmacies in your area, see the Resource Section beginning on page 255.

## SUMMING IT UP

Hormone replacement therapy is a powerful therapeutic tool for staving off all manner of age-related conditions. Like many of the other natural therapies discussed in this book, rejuvenating hormones nourish the brain, improve mental function, and enhance many aspects of general health.

STEP 10

# Strengthen Memory With Smart Drugs and Nutrients

*Mark is founder and CEO of a rapidly growing corporation. He works long hours, oversees dozens of employees, fields scores of telephone calls, and reviews stacks of financial and technical papers every day. His brain is always in overdrive. Mark himself admits (and those around him will agree) that he has a quick temper and a short attention span. It's been a problem all his life, but he has never been able to get it under control—until I introduced him to Dilantin. Now that he takes small doses of this "smart drug" regularly, he finds that his ability to attend to important tasks and screen out interruptions has increased dramatically. This has been accompanied by significant improvements in productivity and interpersonal relationships.*

Smart drugs. Don't you just love that name? This is an actual class of drugs and nutrients known as *nootropics* (literally, "acting on the mind"). Nootropics act on the brain to enhance perception, concentration, cognition, language, and memory. They have been studied in well-controlled clinical trials, and their safety and effectiveness have been repeatedly demonstrated. Millions of people worldwide—those with serious cognitive problems and others who are looking to gain a mental edge—take nootropics. While gaining momentum among patients and medical practitioners in Europe and other parts of the world, nootropics have been virtually ignored by physicians in the United States. Why?

I believe that since memory and cognitive problems generally strike older people, most doctors calmly accept these and other signs of degeneration as the results of normal aging. Normal? According to current standards maybe, but these conditions certainly are not inevitable. The biochemical processes that cause the breakdowns associated with aging have been clearly defined, as

seen in Chapter 2, and solutions for slowing down these processes are readily available. Idly watching patients deteriorate when
we have so many useful tools to retard the process of aging is, in
my opinion, unconscionable.

Second, the entire structure of medical education is so steeped
in disease management that it rarely considers health. What I mean
is that medical students are taught how to recognize and treat illness, but rarely are they instructed in learning how to help patients
achieve optimal health. "If it ain't broken, don't fix it." Well, I disagree. I believe we can improve upon normal function and perhaps
in the process raise the expectations of what "normal" means.

Third, conventional physicians treat patients with drugs and
surgery, period. Sure, they give lip service to exercise and diet
and may give patients the okay to take a one-a-day type of multivitamin, but drugs and surgery are the primary therapies of
conventional medicine. Many nootropics, on the other hand, are
not traditional pharmaceutical drugs. Some are herbal extracts,
others are nutrients—and those that are prescription drugs are
often not recognized for their cognitive-enhancing benefits, or
they are not even available in this country. The prejudice towards
conventional pharmaceutical drugs runs fast and deep throughout the medical profession.

However, I feel the winds of change stirring. We are on the
cusp of a huge demographic shift in this country. Every seven
seconds a baby boomer turns fifty. I predict that as the mass of
well-informed and politically active baby boomers move through
their fifties and sixties, smart drugs and nutrients will become
more and more commonplace. Someday, physician-prescribed
nootropics to perk up flagging mental function may be as prevalent as anti-inflammatory medications prescribed for the aches
and pains of arthritis.

Dozens of compounds have been branded as nootropics, but
I want to tell you about the ones I consider the most powerful. I
do not expect you to run out and immediately add these smart
drugs and nutrients to your regimen. I suggest you first incorporate the diet, nutritional supplements, physical and mental exercise, and recommendations for stress management and sleep
detailed in the first eight steps of this 10-step program. If you are

over age forty-five, look into the hormones described in Step 9. As for the smart drugs and nutrients, I recommend them for two groups. The first group includes those who really need a memory boost, whose cognitive problems are apparent and interfere with their daily lives. If you fall into this category or if you are reading this book to pick up ideas to help a friend or loved one, you should consider one or more of these heavy hitters right away.

Others who will benefit from smart drugs and nutrients consist of those for whom mental sharpness and a keen memory are an absolute requisite for professional or personal reasons. Individuals in this group tend to be proactive about their health. If you fall into this category, you already may be on a preventive program of exercise and nutritional supplements. You may even be taking some of the targeted brain-boosting agents discussed in earlier chapters. Your memory deficits are likely minor and noticeable only to you, but you're concerned and demand the best, most innovative resources available. You're not afraid to try something out of the ordinary. You would be a perfect candidate for a nootropic, even if you only used it periodically during times of mental overload or when peak performance is crucial.

Specific guidelines for selecting and using these remarkable agents are presented at the end of this chapter. If your physician is willing to work with you in implementing these therapies, so much the better. If he or she is not, you might consider finding one who will—the Resource Section beginning on page 255 provides referral information as well as details on how to order prescription drugs from offshore sources.

But first, let me tell you about nine smart drugs and nutrients that are among the most powerful brain protectors and memory boosters in the world.

## CALM DOWN AND FOCUS WITH DILANTIN

We are electrical beings. Down to the cellular level we run on electricity. And our brains are hotbeds of electrical activity. Electrical impulses initiate the release of neurotransmitters at the synapses where dendrites and axons communicate, and electricity moves nerve impulses along throughout the brain. The brain's electrical system occasionally gets out of whack, due to disease, trauma, drug or toxin exposure, or imbalances in brain chemicals. The most dramatic manifestation of this is a seizure. One of the most effective anti-seizure drugs is Dilantin (phenytoin), which was discovered over sixty years ago and remains a staple in conventional pharmacology. However, Dilantin has been found to have much broader therapeutic potential than merely treating seizures.

Low doses of Dilantin have been studied in conjunction with over 100 diseases. It has been found to be especially useful in improving concentration, response time, mental performance, and mood. Most remarkably, it has been shown to raise IQ. Twenty volunteer hospital employees were given the Wechsler IQ test. They were given Dilantin, and then they took the test again. All participants had improvements in overall IQ scores, with the most significant improvements in tests of verbal performance. Jack Dreyfus, the "Lion of Wall Street," a financier who made a fortune in the stock market in the 1960s and founded the Dreyfus Fund, is largely responsible for the solid body of research on this remarkable drug. He was plagued with severe attacks of anxiety, depression, and an inability to function that almost destroyed his career until he came upon Dilantin. Jack was so impressed with how it turned his life around that he set up a foundation—which he has funded to the tune of $70 million—to research Dilantin and educate physicians on its benefits.

Dilantin is believed to enhance cognitive function because of its ability to improve concentration by normalizing the electrical activity in the brain. As Jack Dreyfus described it in his book, *A Remarkable Medicine Has Been Overlooked*, his brain was like a "bunch of dry twigs. It seemed that a thought of fear or anger would light the dry twigs, the fire would spread out of control, and the thoughts couldn't be turned off. Dilantin seemed to act like a gentle rain on the twigs, and the fire (and thoughts) could be kept under control." Jack's description is an apt one, and it indicates the kind of people who benefit most from this drug—people who have concentration difficulties and are unfocused, easily distracted, short-tempered, obsessive and impulsive, and have memory and cognitive problems because of these characteristics. Mark, whose story I opened this chapter with, was like a string of firecrackers, jumping from one unfinished thought to another, until he cooled down his brain with Dilantin.

In my medical practice I probably prescribe Dilantin more than any other nootropic. It has tremendous potential for enhancing memory and mental function, but it is rarely prescribed for this. Most doctors are familiar only with its use in controlling seizures.

Dilantin's patent has expired, so there is no financial incentive for any drug company to pursue it and instruct physicians in its usage. You yourself may have to educate your physician about this drug. Dilantin requires a prescription. The recommended dose is 100 milligrams one to three times a day, which is much less than the dose given for seizures. At this low dose it is quite safe, neither addictive nor sedative, and it has none of the negative side effects that higher doses may have.

## PIRACETAM FACILITATES BRAIN COMMUNICATION

Another of my favorite nootropics is piracetam. I am not alone in my enthusiasm for this smart drug. One single brand of piracetam, Nootropil, registered sales of over $1 billion in recent years. Piracetam raises levels of acetylcholine, the most important neurotransmitter for memory and learning. In addition, it increases the brain's energy reserves and protects it against oxygen starvation. And as convincingly demonstrated in dozens of studies, piracetam also improves mental performance.

One study examined the effects of piracetam on eighteen subjects, fifty years old and older, who were fully functional, worked in demanding jobs, and had above-average IQs but were having problems retaining and recalling information. These are symptoms of age-associated memory impairment, which affects many people once they hit their forties. These volunteers were given tests of cognitive function to measure the speed and efficiency at which they were able to do the following tasks: locate dot patterns on a page, translate digits into corresponding symbols, and order in sequence numbers and letters that had been randomly placed around a circle. They were then divided into two groups; one took piracetam while the other took a placebo. When they were retested, the people taking piracetam scored dramatically higher than the placebo group on all tests. The study was then "crossed over." This means the group that had been taking a placebo was placed on piracetam, and those formerly on piracetam were given a placebo. (This was a double-blind study. No one, including the researchers, knew who got the placebo and who got piracetam until the end of the study.) When the volunteers were tested a final time, once again the scores of the people on piracetam improved, while those taking the placebo declined dramatically.

In another study, piracetam actually improved driving skills. This double-blind, placebo-controlled study, conducted in Germany, tested the skills of 101 older drivers, who were then supplemented with piracetam or a placebo for six weeks. When they were tested again—in real traffic—the drivers taking piracetam displayed significant improvements in traffic observance and sign recognition. Piracetam has also been observed to slow the progression of Alzheimer's disease. Patients with early Alzheimer's disease were given 8 grams of piracetam per day and followed for one year. Compared to the placebo group, the subjects taking piracetam had notably less mental decline over that year. Another study reported results on the combination of piracetam with choline (a B-complex vitamin relative discussed in Steps 2 and 4), which was administered to ten patients with Alzheimer's disease for seven days. Although not all patients benefited from this protocol, three of the ten patients had remarkable enhancements, with a 70-percent improvement on tests of verbal memory after taking piracetam.

An interesting aspect of piracetam's mode of action is that it improves communication across the corpus callosum, which connects the two hemispheres of the brain. Many activities, including speech and cognition, require communication between the right and left brain. Piracetam is helpful in dyslexia, speech disorders, aphasia (inability to express or comprehend properly through speech), and language acquisition in children and adults with Down syndrome—possibly because it helps the right and left hemispheres "talk" to each other. Children with attention deficit disorder have also noticed improvements in focus and attention span while taking piracetam.

Piracetam is an excellent choice for a first step into the world of nootropics. It is exceptionally safe and has no side effects, even at very high doses. It usually comes in 800-milligram capsules, and the recommended dose is 3 to 6 capsules per day (2,400 to 4,800 milligrams). I generally recommend that my patients start out at the higher dose for several days so they can experience piracetam's full effects, then settle into a lower dose, perhaps three 800-milligram capsules per day. If results are not obtained at the lower dose, go back up to 4,800 milligrams. Piracetam is available by prescription in the United States but may be obtained for personal use from overseas without a prescription.

## SLOW BRAIN AGING WITH ACETYL-L-CARNITINE

Acetyl-l-carnitine (ALC) is a derivative of carnitine, an important nutrient that facilitates the transport of fat into the mitochondria where it is metabolized for energy. ALC does truly extraordinary things in the brain. It improves communication among neurons by increasing levels of the neurotransmitter acetylcholine. In fact, ALC actually mimics acetylcholine, as its chemical structure is remarkably similar to that of the neurotransmitter. It also boosts the production of nerve growth factor (NGF) which, as explained in Step 5, stimulates the formation of dendrites. In addition, ALC helps maintain the nerves' protective myelin sheaths and increases the activity of dopamine, a neurotransmitter that stimulates the brain.

ALC also protects your brain from the ravages of aging. It neutralizes free radicals, stabilizes cellular membranes, and boosts flagging energy production in aging brain cells. ALC has proven to be effective in slowing down the progression of Alzheimer's disease. In a 1991 study, 130 patients with Alzheimer's disease were treated with ALC or a placebo and followed for one year. During that time both groups worsened, but those taking ALC had a slower rate of deterioration in thirteen of fourteen categories, including logical intelligence, long-term verbal memory, and selective attention. Another study examined elderly people with less severe mental impairment. The 236 subjects in this study were experiencing mild memory loss and cognitive declines, and supplementing with 1,500 milligrams of ALC resulted in significant improvements in tests measuring memory and constructional thinking.

This smart nutrient also improves mental function in healthy individuals. Italian researchers gave seventeen men and women between the ages of twenty-two and twenty-seven 1,500 milligrams of ALC daily. Study participants were tested for attention levels, hand-eye coordination, and reflexes before starting on the supplement, and then again after thirty days. Reflexes markedly quickened on ALC, as did task completion time. In addition, participants made fewer errors.

The recommended dose for ALC is 500 to 1,500 milligrams per day, in divided doses. I suggest starting at 500 milligrams and gradually increasing the dosage if you don't notice improvements. ALC does not require a prescription and is sold in health food stores. Although its close relative l-carnitine is an important nutritional supplement in its own right, it is not as easily able to cross the blood-brain barrier, and its role in brain health has not been established. It's best to stick with ALC.

## DMAE IMPROVES ATTENTION

Dimethyl-aminoethanol (DMAE) is a natural substance present in foods such as anchovies and sardines (another reason fish is called brain food). It enhances memory and cognitive function by stimulating the production of choline, which, in turn, revs up the synthesis of acetylcholine. DMAE was commonly used prior to the 1980s and was especially effective in children with learning or behavioral problems associated with shortened attention spans and/or hyperactivity (what we now term attention deficit disorder). In one study, Dr. Carl Pfeiffer of the Brain-Bio Center in Princeton, New Jersey, gave 108 children with this behavior profile supplemental DMAE. Improvement was observed in 71 percent of the hyperactive children in the areas of increased attention span, decreased irritability, scholastic improvement, and, in some children, a rise in IQ.

## Using Memory Aids

Below is a list of common aids that can help you remember things. If you aren't already using these tried and true methods, consider incorporating them into your daily life now.

- Writing "to do" lists.

- Making out shopping lists.

- Keeping a journal or diary.

- Tying string around one's finger.

- Keeping a calendar or daily planner.

- Rhyming things to remember *(for example, "In fourteen ninety-two, Columbus sailed the ocean blue")*.

- Creating "letter" memory aids *(for example, the letters of the name "ROY G. BIV" contain the first letters of the colors of the rainbow)*.

- Turning numbers into letters *(to remember information such as telephone numbers—for example, dialing 563–7227 is the same as dialing "JOE'S BAR")*.

DMAE is also useful for adults with cognitive complaints. A 1996 German study examined the effects of DMAE along with vitamins and minerals on sixty men and women between the ages of forty and sixty-five who had difficulty concentrating during mental exercises. In this study, researchers obtained EEG recordings of volunteers before they began taking DMAE or a placebo, and again after twelve weeks of supplementation. There were no changes in the brain waves of the subjects taking the placebo. In those taking DMAE, however, improvements were seen in the frontal and temporal lobes, areas of the brain that play an important role in attention, memory, and flexibility in thinking.

DMAE is sold over the counter in health food stores. Effective doses of DMAE vary from person to person, so start low at 100 milligrams and gradually increase this amount, if necessary, to 300 milligrams. DMAE can cause sleepiness, headaches, and muscle aches in some people when taken in high doses. It is not recommended for patients with epilepsy and bipolar disorder. If you find that you have insomnia while taking DMAE, cut back on the dosage. It is important to note that vitamin B$_5$ (pantothenic acid) must be present for the synthesis of acetylcholine. I suggest taking 50 milligrams of vitamin B$_5$ per day.

## CITICOLINE ENHANCES NEUROTRANSMITTER PRODUCTION

Yet another nootropic that increases levels of acetylcholine is citicoline (cytidine-5'-diphosphocholine). This naturally occurring substance provides the brain with the raw materials it needs for two important brain compounds. The first is choline, which, as you have seen, is an important precursor for the manufacture of acetylcholine. The other is cytidine—a compound that, along with choline, is required for the formation of phosphatidyl choline (PC), one of the primary components of nerve cell membranes. (See Step 3 for an in-depth discussion of PC.)

A number of clinical studies have examined citicoline's effects on the brain. In addition to increasing production of both PC and acetylcholine, citicoline also boosts levels of dopamine and other neurotransmitters. Furthermore, citicoline enhances bioelectrical activity in the brain and protects brain cells from hypoxia (inadequate oxygen) and ischemia (decreased blood flow). It has been successfully used as a treatment for victims of mild to moderate head injuries and concussions, and for patients who have had strokes.

Citicoline has also been demonstrated to improve memory and learning. In a study of twenty-four elderly people with age-related memory deficits, 300 to 1,000 milligrams per day of citicoline significantly improved word recall. A larger study conducted in Spain involved 2,817 people ranging in age from sixty to eighty with symptoms of insufficient blood flow to the brain. In these patients citicoline not only improved memory but also helped depression, insomnia, headaches, and dizziness. In another study—a double-blind trial of ninety-five people between the ages of fifty and eighty-five with some memory problems—the effects of citicoline were compared with a placebo. During the first ninety days of the trial, the subjects with relatively poorer memories taking 1,000 milligrams of citicoline had improvements in delayed recall, compared to the placebo group. The groups were then switched and 2,000 milligrams of citicoline was administered for sixty days. At the higher dosage, not only did the people with poorer memories improve (and more significantly than on the lower dose), but those with relatively intact memories did better on tests of immediate and delayed memory.

The recommended dosage of citicoline is 500 to 1,000 milligrams per day. This may be increased to 2,000 milligrams if symptoms warrant. Citicoline does not require a prescription and is well tolerated at the suggested doses.

## ENERGIZE YOUR BRAIN WITH DEPRENYL

Dopamine is a neurotransmitter that stimulates the brain. Oliver Sacks, M.D., shares an extraordinary story that illustrates the power of this neurotransmitter in his book, *Awakenings*, which was also made into a movie. *Awakenings* is the true story of a group of patients who were in a trancelike state for years until Dr. Sacks gave them massive doses of l-dopa, a drug that is converted into dopamine. After taking this drug, the patients suddenly awoke and temporarily began to function normally.

Levels of dopamine, which also regulates motor control and sex drive, decrease with age. This is partially attributed to the age-related degeneration of a tiny area of your brain called the *substantia nigra*, where an abundance of dopamine-containing neurons abide. Extreme degeneration of the substantia nigra results in Parkinson's disease, a neurological disorder characterized by trembling and loss of muscle control. Another reason for the decline in dopamine levels is that the breakdown of this neurotransmitter, which is facilitated by the enzyme monoamine oxidase (MAO), outstrips its production as we age. The resulting decrease in one of your brain's primary stimulants causes many aspects of brain function to slow down.

A group of drugs has been designed specifically to block or slow down the action of the enzyme that degrades dopamine. Known as MAO inhibitors, these drugs cause a rise in dopamine levels. Among the safest of these drugs is deprenyl. It is known as a type-B MAO inhibitor, meaning that it inhibits MAO activity primarily in the glial cells of the brain, as opposed to the type-A MAO inhibitors that affect cells throughout your body and can raise blood pressure. Deprenyl has many therapeutic uses, including treatment of Parkinson's disease and Alzheimer's disease. A National Institutes of Health study demonstrated improvements in memory, attention, and learning in patients with Alzheimer's disease who were taking 10 milligrams of deprenyl daily.

People who simply want to sharpen their memory also use deprenyl, which is presently being explored as an anti-aging drug. In animal studies, it increased average life span by 40 percent!

Deprenyl is available by prescription under the trade name Eldepryl. However, I prefer liquid deprenyl citrate because it is easier to administer a variety of doses in liquid form. Dosing is age dependent. A daily dose of 1 or 2 milligrams is suggested for people in their forties, with a 1 milligram increase every five years. Therefore, a fifty-five-year-old would take 3 milligrams daily, a sixty-year-old 4 milligrams, and so on. Patients with Alzheimer's disease are recommended to take 5 to 10 milligrams daily. Regardless of age, it's best to start low and build up slowly. Deprenyl is quite safe, although high doses may result in insomnia and irritability in some people. Liquid deprenyl citrate is made by Discovery Experimental and Development, Inc., and is available without a prescription (see the Resource Section beginning on page 255).

## HYDERGINE PROTECTS NEURONS

The mostly widely used prescription drug for improving brain function in Europe is Hydergine. This drug (also called ergoloid mesylates) is extracted from the ergot fungus that grows on rye plants. It is perhaps the most widely studied of the smart drugs. Hydergine improves blood flow in the brain and protects against free-radical damage. It also revs up brain metabolism; increases the production of the stimulating neurotransmitters dopamine and norepinephrine; and decreases the activity of MAO, the enzyme that breaks down dopamine. Furthermore, it may enhance the effects of nerve growth factor and promote the growth of dendrites. Hydergine appears to undo damage to injured brain cells. It is routinely administered in Europe to patients who have suffered a stroke, shock, drug overdose, severe accident, or any other condition that may lead to brain damage.

Hydergine has been intensively studied for the treatment of senile dementia, which is characterized by confusion, memory loss, forgetfulness, depression, dizziness, decreased alertness, mood swings, and/or coordination problems. These symptoms are similar to those of cerebral vascular insufficiency, which is mentioned in the discussion of *Ginkgo biloba* in Step 3, and for good reason. Senile dementia is in large part caused by cerebral vascular insufficiency, or inadequate blood flow and delivery of oxygen and nutrients to the brain. It is believed that Hydergine benefits patients with this type of dementia by improving blood flow and protecting the brain from the free-radical damage caused by insufficient oxygen. In a 1994 study, researchers from the University of Southern California School of Medicine examined forty-seven clinical trials in which Hydergine was used in the treatment of senile dementia. The majority of these trials demonstrated that Hydergine was more effective than a placebo in relieving symptoms of dementia. However, improvements in patients with Alzheimer's disease were minimal.

Hydergine's effectiveness as a brain booster has also been examined in healthy people. In one English study, ten healthy volunteers were administered tests of cognitive function. Then they were given 12 milligrams of Hydergine daily for two weeks. At the end of that period they were retested, and significant improvements were noted in alertness and cognitive function.

The most effective dose of Hydergine in the majority of clinical studies was 9 milligrams (3 milligrams three times a day). It is nontoxic, and the only side effects noted are rare gastrointestinal upset and headaches, which can usually be avoided by starting at a low dose and gradually increasing it. It may take several weeks before Hydergine's effects are noticed. Available in the United States by prescription, Hydergine can also be obtained from offshore sources (see the Resource Section beginning on page 255).

## OXYGENATE YOUR BRAIN WITH VINPOCETINE

Another effective plant-derived nootropic is vinpocetine. This herbal extract comes from the lesser periwinkle (*Vinca minor*). Utilized in Asia and Europe for over twenty years, vinpocetine has only recently become available in the United States. Vinpocetine improves blood flow, circulation, and oxygen utilization in the brain. It also protects neurons from the devastating effects of disrupted oxygen delivery. It is, therefore, a useful therapy for symptoms of senile dementia and cerebral vascular insufficiency. Researchers at the University of Surrey in England administered either a high or low dose of vinpocetine or a placebo to 203 patients with mild to moderate dementia. Significantly greater improvements were observed in cognitive performance and overall quality of life in the patients taking vinpocetine compared to the placebo group. Interestingly, there was little difference in the degree of improvement between those taking the high and low doses of the herb.

Vinpocetine also steps up energy production in brain cells. It has been studied as a memory booster for young, healthy people, in whom it has been shown to improve short-term memory. In addition, it appears to have anticonvulsant properties. A Russian study of epileptic patients demonstrated that vinpocetine reduced the frequency and, in some cases, completely eliminated epileptic seizures in twenty of the thirty-one patients involved in the study. This nontoxic herbal extract was well tolerated in the bulk of participants in all the clinical studies.

Vinpocetine is sold in health food stores. The recommended dose is 10 milligrams daily. I highly recommend this up-and-coming supplement for improved brain function.

## HUPERZINE A—BRAIN BOOSTER FROM CHINA

Huperzine A is an extract from club moss (*Huperzia serrata*) that has been used in Chinese medicine for centuries to treat inflammation and fever. In recent years, interest in this extract has shifted to its effects on the brain. Huperzine A blocks the enzyme acetylcholinesterase, which breaks down the vital neurotransmitter acetylcholine, and has been demonstrated in clinical studies to enhance focus, concentration, and memory. For patients with Alzheimer's disease and serious dementia, this herbal extract may actually take the place of prescription drugs.

In one study carried out in China, fifty patients with Alzheimer's disease were given 200 micrograms of Huperzine A in four divided doses, and fifty-three other patients with similar degrees of dementia were administered a placebo. Fifty-eight percent of the patients treated with the herb had improvements in memory, cognitive function, and behavior, compared to 36 percent who improved on the placebo.

Interestingly, two of the pharmaceutical drugs approved by the FDA for the treatment of Alzheimer's disease, tacrine (Cognex) and donepezil (Aricept), act in a manner similar to Huperzine A (see the inset on page 224). They inhibit the breakdown of acetylcholine. However, according to an article published in the March 12, 1997, issue of the *Journal of the American Medical Association*, Huperzine A does so in a more natural and elegant way, fitting into the molecule as opposed to "jamming" it up. The herb also has fewer side effects and its actions are of longer duration than the drugs.

In addition to maintaining acetylcholine levels, Huperzine A also protects neurons from the toxic effects of excess glutamate, an excitatory neurotransmitter. The recommended dose of Huperzine A is 200 micrograms per day in divided doses. No prescription is required for this herbal remedy. At this time, I recommend Huperzine A only for patients with Alzheimer's disease or moderate to severe dementia.

## COMMONLY ASKED QUESTIONS ABOUT NOOTROPICS

*Do I really need to take any of these smart drugs and nutrients?*

If you are experiencing minor age-associated memory impairment with an occasional memory slip-up or problems concentrating now and then, I recommend that you initially concentrate on the first eight steps of this 10-step program—diet, physical and mental exercise, stress management, improved sleep, and a broad range of supplemental vitamins, minerals, essential fats,

## Conventional Drugs for Memory Impairment

Most of the conventional FDA-approved drugs for Alzheimer's disease inhibit the action of acetylcholinesterase—the enzyme that breaks down acetylcholine—leaving more of this neurotransmitter available for use by the brain. Acetylcholine is involved in processing memory, and abnormalities in levels and utilization of acetylcholine are central to Alzheimer's disease. The most common prescription drug of this class is tacrine (Cognex). It helps some patients but often causes side effects of nausea, vomiting, sweating, and salivation. Tacrine also has some liver toxicity. A newer, similar drug, which is less toxic to the liver but has similar side effects, is donepezil (Aricept). The herbal extract Huperzine A also inhibits acetylcholinesterase and appears to be a superior alternative to both of these drugs.

Other drugs are in the approval process, and some of them look promising. However, they all address quite severe memory impairment and Alzheimer's disease. Those of you hoping to give your memory a boost and hone your mental edge are better off following the 10-step program.

and herbs. If after three months you feel as if you need an additional boost, consider adding one of the specialized agents discussed in this chapter. On the other hand, if your memory and cognitive complaints are more pressing, I recommend adding one or more of the nootropics right away. If you are caring for someone with severe memory loss or Alzheimer's disease, you should start that person on a comprehensive program that encompasses all ten steps, including nootropics.

### Which nootropics are best for me?

Each smart drug or nutrient addresses slightly different aspects of cognitive decline. Therefore, you should tailor your program to your specific symptoms and needs. Table 4.5 presents a brief overview of the indications for nootropics.

## Is it okay to take nootropics with other memory-enhancing agents?

It is perfectly safe and highly recommended to take nootropics with other memory-enhancing agents discussed in this book. In fact, because the vitamins and minerals, herbs, targeted supplements, and nootropics address a variety of degenerative mechanisms, they work well together to cover all the bases. Taking more than one nootropic is also acceptable.

TABLE 4.5. NOOTROPIC RECOMMENDATIONS

| Symptoms | Recommended Nootropic | Suggested Daily Dosage |
|---|---|---|
| General poor memory | Piracetam, Acetyl-l-carnitine, DMAE, *or* Vinpocetine | • 2,400–4,800 milligrams • 500–1,500 milligrams • 100–300 milligrams • 10 milligrams |
| Problems with attention span and focus | DMAE *or* Dilantin | • 100–300 milligrams • 100–300 milligrams |
| Impulsive or obsessive thoughts that get in the way of clear thinking | Dilantin | • 100–300 milligrams |
| Feeling of mental slowdown and lack of brain energy | Deprenyl *or* Acetyl-l-carnitine | • 1–10 milligrams • 500–1,500 milligrams |
| Signs of cerebral insufficiency, memory loss, plus depression and perhaps dizziness | Hydergine *or* Vinpocetine *or* Citicoline | • 9 milligrams • 10 milligrams • 500–1,000 milligrams |
| Alzheimer's disease or moderate to severe dementia | Huperzine A | • 200 micrograms |

*Where can I find these smart drugs and nutrients?*

Some of these smart nutrients—DMAE, acetyl-l-carnitine, Huperzine A, and vinpocetine—do not require a prescription. They are sold in health food stores and by mail order. See the Resource Section beginning on page 255 for mail order contacts. Others—Dilantin, piracetam, deprenyl, and Hydergine—may be prescribed by your physician. If your physician is unwilling to write a prescription for these drugs, you have two choices. You can either find a more open-minded physician who will work with you or purchase these drugs yourself from offshore companies. It is perfectly legal to order drugs for your own personal use in this manner.

## SUMMING IT UP

This chapter has only scratched the surface of this broad and fascinating category of nootropics. The Resource Section, beginning on page 255, provides a list of recommended books, newsletters, and websites that contain additional information on these smart drugs and nutrients. It also provides information on doctor referrals and where to purchase nootropics.

# CHAPTER 5

---

# Tying It All Together

*A*lice attended the one-week Back to Health program at Whitaker Wellness Institute with her son, James, who came primarily to accompany his mother. He was concerned about her health—she was depressed, forgetful, and becoming increasingly frustrated over her forgetfulness. During their first day at the clinic, Alice and James underwent extensive evaluations with a staff physician. Alice had a long history of hypertension, arthritis, and fibromyalgia, and she showed the doctor her bag filled with the various medications she was taking. James, on the other hand, was a healthy fifty-year-old with no real physical problems.

Both Alice and James were placed on a comprehensive multivitamin and mineral regimen that included high doses of antioxidants and B-complex vitamins, along with essential fatty acids. Alice was also given Ginkgo biloba, phosphatidyl serine, daily vitamin $B_{12}$ injections, and extra vitamin E, as well as St. John's wort to address her depression. She was also taking targeted therapies for her other medical problems. Her physician examined her medications, determined that two of them might be causing some of her symptoms and recommended a plan to reduce or eliminate the likely offenders. James' treatment program was simpler. Because his testosterone level was low for his age, he was started on supplemental testosterone along with a multinutrient program.

Alice and James spent the rest of the week with the other patients and their companions. They dined on nutritious, low-fat, gourmet meals prepared by our chef in a private dining room at the first-class, full-serv-

*ice hotel in which they stayed. They participated in an exercise class every day and took walks in the evening. James attended the daily lectures given by the physicians and professional staff on nutrition, exercise, stress reduction, nutritional supplementation, and alternative approaches to a number of common conditions. As the week progressed and she started feeling better, Alice joined in as well. Together they had a consultation with our certified nutritionist who worked out individualized meal plans for Alice and James.*

*When Alice saw her doctor again later in the week for her second evaluation, she was much more alert and animated. She was appreciative of all the support she had received from the staff and other patients, and was delighted with the improvements in her memory. James confided to her doctor that he had not seen his mother in such good spirits in months—she was like her old self. And he had to admit that he was also feeling more energetic and thinking more clearly. They left for home recharged and motivated with the specific tools they needed to improve their mental and physical health.*

Alice and James are typical of the patients who go through the Back to Health program at the Whitaker Wellness Institute in Newport Beach, California. For many, it is a life-changing week. They lose weight, their blood pressure comes down, and their blood sugar levels normalize. Some may find relief from arthritic pain, allergies, or gastrointestinal distress. But one comment we hear repeatedly from patients at the end of this program— regardless of what their most pressing medical problems are—is that they have more energy, focus, and mental clarity. In some patients, we can attribute this to one specific therapy. A patient with very low vitamin $B_{12}$ levels, for example, might perk right up after two $B_{12}$ injections. Another might respond to a specific herb or smart drug.

However, I am convinced that the majority of patients who experience improvements in memory and cognitive function have benefited from the whole ball of wax. The optimal diet, daily exercise, mental stimulation, stress reduction, and adequate sleep—plus being on an individualized program of nutritional supplements with, perhaps, the addition of hormones or smart drugs—makes the difference. The point is, these patients didn't just clean up their diets or take vitamins or begin to exercise. They did *all* of these things and more. They followed most of the recommendations of the 10-step program for a sharper memory and mental edge.

We've covered a lot of ground in this book. If you've stayed with me this far, congratulations! You've undoubtedly sprouted new dendrites and have made new neuronal connections by learning this information. We've explored the mysteries of the brain, cleared up common misconceptions regarding memory and cognitive function, and—I hope—buried forever the myth that "normal" aging involves memory loss and senility. You are now aware of the factors that put your brain at risk, and you know how to avoid these risks and reduce your likelihood of problems down the line.

But the heart and soul of this book lies in the ten specific, time-tested, patient-proven steps for improving your memory and cognitive function, regardless of your age. You've read them—you may even know them by heart—but they aren't going to do you any good unless you implement them. So let's get started.

## ONE STEP AT A TIME

While I've organized this 10-step program in what I consider to be the most logical order, these steps can be approached from almost any direction. Those who are more "left-brained" and analytical will probably prefer to begin with Step 1. Others may want to start with the step that seems easiest, or the one they feel offers the most punch. Simply start somewhere, and proceed at your own pace. As the old saying goes, the longest journey begins with a single step.

## EVALUATE YOUR PROGRESS

Evaluating your progress on this program presents something of a challenge. Unlike with weight loss, you can't measure improvements in memory on a scale, nor is there a blood test that determines cognitive function. One way to track your progress is by keeping a journal. This journal doesn't have to be elaborate—just make daily entries about what measures you're taking to improve your memory and mental edge, how you're feeling, and what changes you've noticed. Rate your feeling of alertness, degree of perception, and performance at work and on intellectual tasks, games, and the like—and write your observations in your journal. I know it's difficult to evaluate your own mental function, but by recording these small observations, trends will emerge.

Feedback from people close to you is also important. One of my patients stated that since she's been taking piracetam, people tell her she's funnier—her sense of humor is more acute. Another reports that since he began working out regularly—going to the gym four times a week—his colleagues feel he's been much better organized. Yet another patient told me that his increased focus and work output, which he attributes to taking Dilantin, have been noticed by his boss.

If you have a computer with access to the Internet, I highly recommend that you visit *http://www.brain.com* and check out the *THINKfast* software offered at this website. *THINKfast* is an interactive tool that gives a composite score of reaction time, perceptual threshold, working memory, and memory capacity. What I like about this program is that it's not any kind of competition—it's just a series of entertaining games and exercises. You create your own baseline by repeating a five-minute test every day for five or ten days until your score is more or less stable. You'll then have something concrete to measure benefits of these various therapies against. Try phosphatidyl serine, for example, for a couple of weeks, and then test yourself. Get serious about exercise for a month, then test again. You'll have a lot of fun with *THINKfast,* and it also provides mental exercise that boosts your brain power. If you enjoy the sample test at the website, you might want to order the software.

## RECAP

Now let's briefly recap the elements of this 10-step program for building and maintaining better memory.

## Step 1—Feed Your Head

Eat a diet of fresh, unprocessed foods, with an emphasis on veg-etables, fruits, whole grains, and legumes. Go easy on starchy carbohydrates, such as breads, potatoes, rice, and most cereals. Include some lean protein with each meal, and make sure you eat fish several times a week (salmon and other cold-water fish are best). Avoid saturated fats from animal sources and processed fats and oils. Do include small amounts of healthy fats such as flaxseed oil. Drink a lot of water, and avoid excess caffeine. Strictly avoid aspartame (NutraSweet) and MSG.

## Step 2—Protect Your Brain with Vitamins and Minerals

Everyone should take a high-potency multivitamin/mineral sup-plement. Make sure it contains adequate amounts of the follow-ing key nutrients for your brain:

| Vitamin/Mineral | Suggested Daily Dosage |
|---|---|
| Vitamin A | 5,000 international units |
| Beta-carotene | 15,000 international units |
| Vitamin $B_1$ (thiamin) | 50 milligrams |
| Vitamin $B_3$ (niacin) | 100 milligrams |
| Vitamin $B_5$ (pantothenic acid) | 50 milligrams |
| Vitamin $B_6$ (pyridoxine) | 75 milligrams |
| Vitamin $B_{12}$ | 100 micrograms |
| Vitamin C | 2,500 milligrams |
| Vitamin E | 800 international units |
| Choline | 425 milligrams* |
| Folic acid | 400 micrograms |
| Magnesium | 500 milligrams |
| Zinc | 30 milligrams |

* 450 milligrams for pregnant women; 550 milligrams for nursing mothers.

If you are over sixty years old or have severe cognitive def-icits, I strongly suggest you get regular injections of 1,000 micrograms of vitamin $B_{12}$ twice a week for one month, then decrease the dosage to twice a month. Taking oral or sublingual doses of vitamin $B_{12}$ daily is another option.

## Step 3—Restore Memory With Herbs

I highly recommend the herb *Ginkgo biloba.* Look for a standardized extract of *Ginkgo biloba* that contains 24-percent ginkgo flavone glycosides and 6-percent terpene lactones. Take 60 milligrams twice a day with meals for a minimum of twelve weeks. (It may take this long to begin to notice effects.) Be aware that ginkgo may react with MAO inhibitor antidepressants and with blood thinners such as warfarin (Coumadin).

## Step 4—Nurture Your Brain With Fats

A basic nutritional supplement program should also include omega-3 fatty acids, especially the "smart fat" docosahexaenoic acid (DHA). The best sources are fish oil capsules (two 1,000-milligram capsules per day—each containing approximately 120 milligrams of DHA), or algae-derived DHA (100 to 200 milligrams daily). Freshly ground flaxseed ($^1/_4$ cup) or flaxseed oil ($1^1/_2$ to 3 tablespoons) is also good.

Try phosphatidyl serine in a dose of 300 milligrams a day for one month, then taper down to 100 milligrams. Also consider 100 to 200 milligrams of phosphatidyl choline daily.

## Step 5—Exercise for Peak Mental Performance

Exercise for a minimum of thirty minutes four times per week to increase the blood flow to your brain and to strengthen the brain itself. Start out slowly and don't overdo it—but make sure you do it.

## Step 6—Sharpen Your Mind With Mental Workouts

Challenge your brain. Read, write, listen to books on tape, learn new words, or memorize favorite poems or passages. Play games, listen to complex music, solve puzzles, master a new subject, or acquire a new skill. Take classes in new areas of interest, travel, or volunteer your time and your talents. Either use your brain or lose it.

## Step 7—Reduce Mind-Numbing Stress

Get your stress level under control by slowing down, eating right, avoiding caffeine, and replenishing vitamins and minerals. (Stress is a known vitamin and mineral depleter.) Physical exercise is a powerful stress reducer, as are listening to music and practicing slow breathing and relaxation exercises. I also recommend the antistress herb ginseng—either 75 to 150 milligrams per day of *Panax ginseng* (standardized for 7-percent ginsenosides), or 75 to 150 milligrams per day of Siberian ginseng (standardized for 0.8-percent eleutherosides). The hormones DHEA and melatonin also combat the effects of stress.

For depression, you might want to try 300 milligrams twice a day of St. John's wort (standardized to contain 0.3-percent hypericin). For anxiety, try 150 milligrams one to six times per day of kava (standardized to contain 30-percent kavalactones).

## Step 8—Rejuvenate Your Brain With Sleep

Eliminate the most common sleep disrupters, including caffeine, nicotine, alcohol, and certain drugs, and create an environment that is conducive to sleep. If you have trouble sleeping, try taking one of the following thirty to forty-five minutes before going to bed: 0.5 to 6 milligrams of melatonin; 50 to 100 milligrams of 5-HTP; or 150 to 300 milligrams of the herb valerian (standardized to contain 0.8-percent valeric acid).

## Step 9—Enhance Brain Function With Hormones

If you are over age forty-five or fifty, I suggest having a hormone analysis done at your doctor's office. If your levels are low, consider hormone replacement therapy. Some hormones are available without a prescription—pregnenolone (50 milligrams per

# Cutting-Edge Therapies for Improved Brain Function

In addition to the nutritional, supplemental, pharmaceutical, hormonal, and lifestyle therapies for the prevention and treatment of mental declines, there are a number of unique cutting-edge approaches as well. Two of them—chelation therapy and enhanced external counterpulsation (EECP)—are unique in concept and powerful in practice. Both have remarkable potential for improving memory and cognition or treating dementia.

## CHELATION THERAPY

Chelation therapy involves the slow administration, via an intravenous infusion, of EDTA—a synthetic protein that binds to and removes heavy metals such as lead and cadmium from the body. It is the treatment of choice for lead poisoning. In fact, its benefits for circulatory and cardiovascular disease were noted almost accidentally when World War II veterans who were being treated for lead toxicity showed striking improvements in atherosclerosis.

Chelation has since been used by tens of thousands of patients for the successful treatment of heart disease, peripheral vascular disease, carotid artery stenosis, and other circulatory problems. It has also been used to treat memory deficits, as it improves circulation in the brain. Few studies have been done on this particular application of chelation therapy, but clinical experience demonstrates that it is a viable treatment for age-associated memory impairment. I do not recommend chelation for patients with moderate or advanced Alzheimer's disease, as the mechanisms causing their mental decline go far beyond impaired circulation.

EDTA chelation must be administered in a doctor's office. An infusion generally lasts about three hours, and the normal course includes twenty to thirty treatments. For a referral to a physician in your area who administers chelation therapy, see the Resource Section beginning on page 255.

---

## ENHANCED EXTERNAL COUNTERPULSATION

Enhanced external counterpulsation (EECP) is a mechanical therapy used primarily for treating cardiovascular disease. Developed at Harvard University in the early 1950s as a treatment for angina pectoris (chest pain associated with blocked coronary arteries), EECP has therapeutic potential for any number of conditions caused by inadequate blood flow—including memory loss.

An EECP treatment involves lying flat on a special bed with what amounts to a body stocking strapped to your lower abdomen and extremities. The body stocking contracts in synchrony with each beat of your heart, forcing blood up the extremities, toward the heart. Blood flow is thus increased to your heart muscle, to your brain, and throughout your body. It's a brilliantly simple concept, and it works. An EECP treatment opens up collateral circulation around blocked vessels and delivers much-needed oxygen.

Your brain requires a constant influx of oxygen. When circulation is impaired within the brain itself or through the carotid arteries that supply blood to the brain, memory and cognitive function are affected. My heart patients who have been through a course of EECP report that their memories have become sharper after treatment. Blood flow to the brain improved so much in one patient that for several hours after every treatment, he could see perfectly without the reading glasses he depended on most of the time.

Although EECP is performed at the Whitaker Wellness Institute, it is not yet widely available. I do, however, foresee this safe, relatively inexpensive therapy becoming more widely used in the near future as insurance companies take a harder look at the costly, dangerous alternatives for vascular diseases.

day), DHEA (25 to 50 milligrams a day for women and 50 to 100 milligrams a day for men), and topical natural progesterone. Estrogen, oral progesterone, thyroid, and testosterone require a prescription. Replacement of these hormones should be discussed with your physician. Insist on natural, human-identical estrogen, progesterone, and testosterone. Also request natural thyroid, if it is needed.

## Step 10—Strengthen Memory With Smart Drugs and Nutrients

Nootropics are powerful substances that can enhance perception, concentration, thought, language, and memory. The ones I recommend most highly are Dilantin, piracetam, acetyl-l-carnitine, DMAE, citicoline, deprenyl, Hydergine, vinpocetine, and Huperzine A.

## BACK TO HEALTH

As you implement the ten steps of this comprehensive program, don't forget that natural therapies are not a quick fix—it may take some time before you notice results, so be patient. However, I am convinced that as you stick with the program and make the suggested positive changes in your life, you will significantly enhance your memory and brain function, as well as your general health and sense of well-being. I applaud you for your desire to improve your health and especially for your willingness to do something about it. You'll find that an improved memory, clearer thinking, and sharper mental edge are well worth it.

# A Final Word

Thinking, perceiving, and remembering are the essence of being human. Whether you have read this book because you or a loved one is experiencing some degree of cognitive decline, or because you just want to be—and continue to be—at your sharpest, I sincerely hope that the suggestions I have presented will help. Use them and soar.

# Glossary

**Acetylcholine.** Neurotransmitter involved in memory and learning; low levels of acetylcholine in the brain are typical in those with Alzheimer's disease.

**Acetyl-l-carnitine (ALC).** Nutritional supplement derived from the amino acid l-carnitine, ALC protects neurons by neutralizing free radicals, stabilizing cellular membranes, boosting the production of nerve growth factor, and enhancing the activity of acetylcholine.

**Adaptogen.** Substance that safely increases resistance to stress and balances body functions. Ginseng is an example of an adaptogen.

**Adrenal gland.** One of two organs situated above the kidneys and comprised of a medulla and cortex. The adrenal medulla produces the hormones epinephrine and norepinephrine, which play a part in controlling heart rate and blood pressure. The adrenal cortex produces steroid hormones that have numerous functions throughout the body.

**Adrenaline.** *See* Epinephrine.

**Advanced glycation end products (AGEs).** Chemically altered proteins formed as a reaction to excess sugar. AGEs can cause damage to the immune, nervous, and endocrine systems. *See also* Glycation.

**Age-associated memory impairment.** Progressive decline in memory and cognitive function, generally beginning between the ages of forty and fifty. This type of memory loss is not to be confused with Alzheimer's disease or other forms of dementia.

**Alarm reaction.** The first phase of the stress response, in which epinephrine and norepinephrine are secreted by the adrenal glands to trigger the metabolic changes of the "fight or flight" response.

**Alpha waves.** Slow, low-amplitude brain waves that indicate a calm, relaxed state of wakefulness.

**Alpha-linolenic acid (ALA).** An essential fatty acid of the omega-3 family that converts to docosahexaenoic acid (DHA) and eicosapentaenoic acid (EPA), which are important for proper brain function.

**Alzheimer's disease.** Progressive type of dementia, characterized by confusion, disorientation, and deterioration of memory, language skills, behavior, and personality. It is not to be confused with age-associated memory impairment.

**Amygdala.** Region of the limbic system that adds emotional color to experiences and memories.

**Andropause.** Gradual decline in testosterone levels that causes loss of muscle mass, as well as reduced libido, energy, and motivation in men around the age of forty-five or fifty. It is similar to the female menopause.

**Antioxidant.** Substance, such as vitamin A, C, or E, or the mineral selenium, that helps protect cells by neutralizing toxic free radicals.

**APOE4.** Variant form of a gene that is used to make the protein apolipoprotein E. It occurs more often in people with Alzheimer's disease than in the general population.

**Apolipoprotein E.** Lipoprotein (fat and protein compound) that carries cholesterol in the blood and appears to play some role in the brain.

**Arachidonic acid (AA).** Omega-6 essential fatty acid that is a structural component of brain cells. When not balanced by other fatty acids, AA can form highly inflammatory and sometimes damaging prostaglandins. It is found in meat, dairy products, and eggs.

**Aspartame (NutraSweet).** Artificial sweetener derived from the amino acids aspartate and phenylalanine. This commonly used food additive overstimulates brain neurons and has been implicated in dizziness, mood changes, vision problems, headaches, and seizures.

**Atherosclerosis.** Narrowing of the arteries and reduction in blood supply due to fatty deposits that thicken the inner layers of the artery walls.

**Axon.** Nerve fiber of a neuron that transmits impulses to the dendrites of another neuron.

**Barbiturate.** Potentially addicting drug that is commonly prescribed to promote sleep. Barbiturates depress respiration, blood pressure, body temperature, and central nervous system activity, and they may cause drowsiness, dizziness, depression, anxiety, irritability, and mental impairment.

**Benzodiazepine.** Class of drugs, including tranquilizers and hypnotics, with strong addiction potential. Adverse reactions include drowsiness, loss of coordination, impaired memory and cognition, and increased aggression and hostility. Abrupt withdrawal may produce seizures and acute psychosis.

**Beta amyloid.** Protein found in dense deposits in the senile plaques and neurofibrillary tangles that are characteristic of Alzheimer's disease.

**Beta waves.** Irregular brain waves that are higher in frequency than alpha waves, and that occur when one is awake and mentally alert.

**Blood-brain barrier.** Dual layer of cells that covers the outside of neurons. It prevents certain drugs, toxins, and disease-causing organisms from making their way to the central nervous system via the bloodstream.

**Brain stem.** Most primitive region of the brain, the brain stem controls heartbeat, circulation, and respiration. Also known as the "reptilian brain."

**Broca's area.** Region of the frontal cortex involved in the production of speech.

**Cell body.** Central portion of a nerve cell that contains the nucleus and is responsible for making proteins and membranes.

**Cerebellum.** Section of the brain that lies just behind the brain stem at the back of the head. It is involved in the central regulation of movement, coordination, muscle tone, and equilibrium.

**Cerebral cortex.** Part of the brain most involved in learning, language, and reasoning. It is comprised of a thin layer that covers the cerebrum. Also called the neocortex.

**Cerebral vascular insufficiency.** Inadequate blood flow to the brain.

**Cerebrovascular accident.** *See* Stroke.

**Cerebrum.** The largest and uppermost portion of the brain, consisting of a right and left hemisphere and crucially involved in thought, emotion, and memory. Also known as the "mammalian brain."

**Chelation.** Procedure in which toxic heavy metals are pulled from the body as the result of an intravenous infusion of the synthetic protein EDTA. This therapy has also been used to help improve circulation in treating vascular disease and memory deficits.

**Cholesterol.** Substance produced by the body or derived from food that is a precursor to steroid hormones. Cholesterol is a crucial component of cell membranes and the myelin sheaths that protect and insulate axons. High levels are associated with an increased risk of heart attack and stroke.

**Choline.** Nutrient that is essential in the manufacture of the neurotransmitter acetylcholine, which plays a crucial role in memory and learning. Supplemental choline may improve memory in some patients with mild to moderate dementia or Alzheimer's disease.

**Circadian rhythm.** Pattern of activity, such as sleep/wakefulness, that is based on a twenty-four hour cycle.

**Citicoline.** Naturally occurring nootropic that helps boost the production of acetylcholine and phosphatidyl choline. Citicoline also enhances electrical activity in the brain, protects brain cells from damage caused by insufficient blood or oxygen, and may improve memory and learning.

**Coenzyme $Q_{10}$ (CoQ$_{10}$).** Nutrient that is essential for energy production in the mitochondria of all cells of the body, including brain cells. It is also a potent antioxidant.

**Corpus callosum.** The band of nerve fibers that connects the right and left cerebral hemispheres.

**Corticosteroid.** Hormone secreted by the adrenal cortex that influences key processes in the body, including metabolism and blood pressure. Chronic stress can result in high levels of corticosteroids that impair immunity and accelerate aging of the brain.

**Cortisol.** Type of cortocosteroid. When chronically elevated, it can cause injury and death to brain cells.

**Dehydroepiandrosterone (DHEA).** Steroid hormone from which estrogen and progesterone may be derived. DHEA enhances immune function and helps counteract the detrimental effects of stress on brain cells. Low levels are associated with cardiovascular disease, obesity, diabetes, cancer, and Alzheimer's disease.

**Delta waves.** Slowest type of brain wave, indicating a state of deep, dreamless sleep.

**Dementia.** Progressive mental disorder characterized by personality disintegration, confusion, disorientation, and impaired cognition and memory. Dementia may be reversible or irreversible, as in the case of Alzheimer's disease.

**Dendrites.** Branch-like extensions of a neuron that receive messages from axons.

**Deprenyl.** Drug that prevents the destruction of the neurotransmitter dopamine. It is used in the treatment of Parkinson's disease, loss of libido, depression, and Alzheimer's disease.

**DHA.** *See* Docosahexaenoic acid.

**DHEA.** *See* Dehydroepiandrosterone.

**Dilantin.** *See* Phenytoin.

**Dimethylaminoethanol (DMAE).** Natural substance that stimulates the production of the neurotransmitter acetylcholine.

**Docosahexaenoic acid (DHA).** Principal fatty acid of the brain, involved in nerve cell communication and memory, and manufactured from dietary or supplemental omega-3 fatty acids. DHA deficiencies are associated with an increased risk of memory loss, dementia, and Alzheimer's disease.

**Dopamine.** Energizing neurotransmitter that affects mood, memory, sex drive, and motor control.

**EDTA chelation.** *See* Chelation.

**Eicosapentaenoic acid (EPA).** Fatty acid that enhances brain function by improving blood flow and delivery of oxygen and nutrients to the brain. EPA is manufactured in the body from dietary or supplemental omega-3 fatty acids.

**Electroencephalograph.** Instrument for recording brain wave activity.

**Endorphins.** Neurotransmitters produced by the brain in response to stress. They reduce the perception of pain and elevate mood.

**Enhanced External Counterpulsation (EECP).** Mechanical therapy in which compression is used to increase blood flow and oxygen supply to the heart, brain, and throughout the body.

**EPA.** *See* Eicosapentaenoic acid.

**Epinephrine.** Chief hormone produced by the adrenal gland that regulates heart rate and metabolism. It helps initiate the "fight or flight" response during periods of stress.

**Ergoloid mesylates.** *See* Hydergine.

**Essential fatty acid (EFA).** Type of polyunsaturated fatty acid required for proper growth, maintenance, and functioning of the body. EFAs are essential to the manufacture of prostaglandins, cell membranes, and myelin sheaths; they can only be obtained from the diet. *See also* Omega-3 fatty acid; Omega-6 fatty acid.

**Estradiol.** Most potent naturally occurring form of human estrogen.

**Estriol.** Relatively weak naturally occurring form of human estrogen.

**Estrogen.** Steroid hormone that promotes the development of female secondary sex characteristics and also plays an important role in bone remodeling, cardiovascular health, and brain function.

**Exhaustion.** Final stage of the stress response in which hormone stores are depleted and organ systems begin to fail.

**"Fight or flight" response.** The body's reaction to a dangerous or threatening situation in which it prepares to stay and fight the danger or run from it.

**Filtering errors.** Lapses in the transfer of information from working memory to long-term memory caused by excessive stimulation from the environment.

**5-hydroxytryptophan (5-HTP).** Precursor to the neurotransmitter serotonin that is used therapeutically as an antidepressant and sleep aid. 5-HTP is synthesized in the body from tryptophan, or derived from the seeds of the West African plant *Griffonia simplicifolia*.

**Free radicals.** Highly reactive molecules that bind to and destroy cellular compounds, including cell membranes, proteins, and DNA.

**Frontal lobe.** Portion of the cerebrum that significantly influences personality and is involved in higher mental activities, including planning, judgment, and abstract reasoning.

**Gamma-aminobutyric acid (GABA).** Calming neurotransmitter that prevents the brain from being overwhelmed by excessive stimulation.

**Gamma-linolenic acid (GLA).** Omega-6 fatty acid that produces protective anti-inflammatory prostaglandins.

**General adaptation system.** *See* Stress response.

*Ginkgo biloba.* Herb with powerful antioxidant properties that can help improve blood circulation and delivery of oxygen and nutrients to the brain.

**Ginseng.** Class of herbs that balance bodily functions and increase physical and mental energy and stamina. Popular types include *Panax ginseng* and Siberian ginseng. *See also* Adaptogen.

**Glial cells.** Brain cells that provide the structural support for neurons. Also called neuroglia.

**Glucocorticoid.** Adrenal hormone such as cortisol. Excessive levels, commonly produced under chronic stress, may be toxic to the brain.

**Glutamate.** Amino acid that acts as an excitatory neurotransmitter in the brain. When balanced with GABA, glutamate helps keep the brain on an even keel.

**Glycation.** Reaction between cellular proteins and excess glucose that results in chemically damaged proteins. It is considered one of the four leading causes of aging. *See also* Advanced glycation end products.

**Glycemic index.** List of values assigned to foods according to the rate at which blood sugar levels rise after they are eaten. A high glycemic index value indicates a food that produces a *rapid* rise in blood sugar, followed by a dramatic fall. A low glycemic index value indicates a food that produces a *gradual* rise and fall in blood sugar.

**Hippocampus.** Region of the limbic system that plays a role in converting new information into long-term memories.

**Homocysteine.** Byproduct of normal amino acid metabolism. High levels can become toxic—impairing circulation, stimulating free-radical damage to cells, and accelerating atherosclerosis, cancer, Alzheimer's, and other degenerative conditions. *See also* Methylation.

**Huperzine A.** Extract from club moss *(Huperzia serrata)* that inhibits the breakdown of the neurotransmitter acetylcholine. It has been demonstrated in clinical studies to enhance concentration and memory.

**Hydergine.** Nootropic widely prescribed in Europe that enhances blood and oxygen supply to the brain, protects against free-radical damage, speeds up brain metabolism, and may enhance the effects of nerve growth factor and promote the growth of dendrites. Also called ergoloid mesylates.

**Hypertension.** Condition in which blood pressure levels are consistently increased. Hypertension often has no symptoms in its earliest stages, but may eventually cause heart attack, congestive heart failure, or stroke.

**Hypothalamus.** Part of the brain's limbic system that regulates blood pressure, heart contractions, respiration, sleep-wake cycles, body temperature, hunger, and thirst. It also controls endocrine system functioning and is the center for emotional response and behavior.

**Hypothyroidism.** Condition caused by the deficient activity of the thyroid gland. Symptoms include lowered metabolic rate, weight gain, and general loss of vigor.

**Hypoxia.** Inadequate supply of oxygen to an organ or body part.

**Inflammation.** Short-lived response by the immune system to tissue injury or invasion by bacteria or other harmful agents that serves to protect the site and promote healing. Chronic inflammation is linked to numerous diseases of aging, including arthritis, cardiovascular disease, dementia, and Alzheimer's disease.

**Insulin.** Hormone secreted by the pancreas to lower blood glucose levels.

**Insulin resistance.** Metabolic disorder in which the body produces adequate insulin but is unable to utilize it correctly to maintain healthy blood glucose levels.

**Ischemia.** Decreased supply of oxygenated blood to an organ or body part.

**Kava.** Herb *(Piper methysticum)* that targets the limbic system to help relieve anxiety and produce a sense of calm and peacefulness without impairing concentration or memory.

**LA.** *See* Linoleic acid.

**Lecithin.** Naturally occurring compound that is rich in phosphatidyl choline, an important component of nerve cell membranes.

**Left hemisphere.** Left side of the cerebrum. This hemisphere controls the right side of the body and is the dominant region for language, mathematical abilities, and logic in the majority of people.

**Limbic system.** Area deep in the brain consisting of the hippocampus, amygdala, hypothalamus, thalamus, and pituitary gland. It mediates emotional responses and is involved in memory processing.

**Linoleic acid (LA).** Essential fatty acid from the omega-6 family.

**Long-term memory.** Durable memory of personal events, knowledge of the world, and procedural knowledge (such as knowing how to drive a car or knit a sweater).

**Medulla.** Portion of the brain stem that contains the cardiovascular and respiratory centers of the brain.

**Melatonin.** Hormone secreted by the pineal gland in response to changes in temperature and light that plays a key role in regulating sleep.

**Menopause.** Gradual decline in levels of estrogen and progesterone that causes the cessation of menstruation. Lowered levels of these hormones have an adverse effect on bone density, cardiovascular health, and cognitive function.

**Methyl donor.** Nutrient such as vitamin $B_{12}$ that contributes a methyl group to a toxic compound in order to neutralize it.

**Methylation.** Body's primary mechanism for neutralizing harmful compounds by combining them with methyl groups. Defects are associated with degenerative diseases, including heart disease, cancer, and Alzheimer's disease. *See also* Homocysteine.

**Microglia.** Supporting cells of the central nervous system that help protect the brain from neural damage and inflammation.

**Monoamine oxidase (MAO) inhibitor.** Drug, such as deprenyl, that raises levels of dopamine by blocking the activity of an enzyme that breaks down this neurotransmitter.

**Monosodium glutamate (MSG).** Food additive that increases levels of the excitatory neurotransmitter glutamate in the brain. It is considered a neurotoxin due to its harmful effects on nerve cells.

**Monounsaturated fat.** Type of fat found in vegetable oils such as olive, canola, and peanut. It is liquid at room temperature and relatively stable when exposed to heat. The body can produce this type of fat.

**Motor cortex.** Functional portion of the cerebrum that conveys signals for action from the brain to the body.

**MSG.** *See* Monosodium glutamate.

**Myelin sheath.** Fatty covering surrounding most nerve fibers that protects and insulates them. It increases the transmission speed of nerve impulses.

**Neocortex.** *See* Cerebral cortex.

**Nerve growth factor (NGF).** Hormone-like protein that promotes the growth, differentiation, and maintenance of neurons.

**Neuroglia.** *See* Glial cells.

**Neuron.** Basic nerve cell of the nervous system composed of a cell body, one or more receptive extensions (dendrites), and a transmitting extension (axon).

**Neurotoxins.** Poisonous substances such as heavy metals, food additives, and certain drugs that can negatively affect the brain and nervous system.

**Neurotransmitter.** Chemical that serves as the basis of communication between nerve cells.

**NGF.** *See* Nerve growth factor.

**Nootropics.** Class of drugs that enhance cognition, memory, concentration, and/or perception.

**Noradrenaline.** *See* Norepinephrine.

**Norepinephrine.** Neurotransmitter and adrenal hormone that helps lay down new memories and transfer memories from short-term to long-term storage in the brain. It also changes blood flow patterns and raises blood pressure during periods of acute stress.

**NREM sleep.** Portion of the sleep cycle consisting of four stages, during which the brain becomes progressively less aware of the environment. This stage precedes and follows each episode of REM sleep.

**NutraSweet.** *See* Aspartame.

**Occipital lobe.** Portion of the cerebrum that governs vision.

**Omega-3 fatty acid.** Type of polyunsaturated fatty acid found in fish oil and flaxseed oil. ALA, DHA, and EPA are types of omega-3 fatty acids.

**Omega-6 fatty acid.** Type of essential fatty acid found in vegetable oils, meats, and dairy products. LA, AA, and GLA are types of omega-6 fatty acids.

**Oxidation.** The generation of highly reactive molecules called free radicals as a consequence of normal cellular processes; these molecules damage cell membranes, proteins, and DNA and accelerate the aging process.

**Paradoxical sleep.** *See* REM sleep.

**Parietal lobe.** Portion of the cerebrum that helps process information that is received from the senses.

**Parkinson's disease.** Degenerative neurological disorder caused by a decrease in brain levels of the neurotransmitter dopamine. It is characterized by muscle tremors, weakness, and shuffling gait.

**Phenytoin (Dilantin).** Anti-seizure medication that is useful in low doses to improve mood, concentration, and general cognitive function.

**Phosphatidyl choline.** Type of phospholipid that is a constituent of nerve cell membranes. It facilitates communication between cells.

**Phosphatidyl serine.** Type of phospholipid that plays a major role in determining the integrity and fluidity of brain cell membranes. It also helps relay chemical messages between neurons, and stimulates the production of the neurotransmitters dopamine, serotonin, and norepinephrine.

**Phospholipid.** A type of fat that forms the chief component of cell membranes and is prevalent in nervous tissue. *See also* Phosphatidyl choline; Phosphatidyl serine.

**Phytochemicals.** Compounds occurring naturally in plant foods that have powerful protective activity in the human body. Examples include lutein in leafy greens, allicin in garlic, and lycopene in tomatoes.

**Pineal gland.** Tiny structure in the brain that secretes melatonin. It is involved in regulating the body clock and influencing reproductive function.

**Piracetam.** Prescription drug that enhances mental function by raising acetylcholine levels, increasing the brain's energy reserves, and improving communication between the right and left hemispheres of the brain.

**Pituitary gland.** Tiny structure found in the brain that functions as a part of both the nervous and endocrine systems. It secretes at least nine major hormones that are involved in a variety of body functions.

**Polyunsaturated fat.** Dietary fat found in fatty fish, vegetable oils, and nut butters, and having a flexible structure and high biological activity. It is a source of essential fatty acids that are crucial for optimal brain function and the formation of cell membranes and prostaglandins.

**Pons.** Portion of the brain stem that provides a link between the upper and lower levels of the central nervous system.

**Pregnenolone.** Precursor hormone from which DHEA, estrogen, testosterone, and other hormones are made. It helps protect nerve cells, enhance memory, and stabilize emotions.

**Progesterone.** Hormone produced by the ovaries that works with estrogen to regulate the menstrual cycle. It is also produced in the central nervous system and stimulates the formation of the nerves' protective myelin sheaths.

**Prostaglandins.** Powerful hormone-like chemical messengers that are produced in most tissues of the body from essential fatty acids. They help regulate nerve transmission, inflammation, blood pressure, heart function, and hormone synthesis.

**REM sleep.** Stage of sleep in which rapid eye movements and dreams occur. Also called paradoxical sleep.

**Reptilian brain.** *See* Brain stem.

**Resistance reaction.** Second phase of the stress response in which levels of cortisol rise dramatically, promoting the breakdown of proteins, elevation of blood pressure, and loss of magnesium, potassium, and other essential nutrients.

**Reticular formation.** Functional region of the brain stem that is responsible for maintaining arousal in the higher brain (the cerebral cortex), relaying significant sensory input to the cortex, and helping to control motor activity.

**Right hemisphere.** Right side of the cerebrum. This hemisphere controls the left side of the body and is the dominant region for visual-spatial skills, facial recognition, intuition, emotion, and the appreciation of art and music in the majority of people.

**St. John's wort.** Herb *(Hypericum perforatum)* used therapeutically to relieve depression. Studies have shown that it works as well as certain prescription antidepressants, without the side effects.

**Saturated fat.** Type of fat found in animal products and tropical oils that has a rigid chemical structure and is solid or semi-solid at room temperature; excess dietary saturated fat promotes obesity and heart disease.

**Selective serotonin reuptake inhibitor (SSRI).** Drug, such as Prozac, that increases levels of circulating serotonin—a neurotransmitter intimately involved in the regulation of mood and sleep. SSRIs have the potential for serious side effects, including suicidal thoughts, restlessness, and aggression.

**Sensory cortex.** Functional portion of the cerebrum in which information from the five senses enters awareness.

**Serotonin.** Neurotransmitter that plays a key role in regulating mood and sleep. Low levels are associated with depression and insomnia.

**Short-term memory.** *See* Working memory.

**Short-wave sleep.** First two stages of NREM sleep that are characterized by high-frequency, low-amplitude brain waves. During this type of sleep, a gradual transition from being awake to being in a light sleep occurs.

**Slow-wave sleep.** Final two stages of NREM sleep that are characterized by low-frequency, high-amplitude brain waves. During this type of sleep, responsiveness to the environment is minimal, and it is difficult to be roused.

**Smart drugs.** *See* Nootropics.

**SSRI.** *See* Selective serotonin reuptake inhibitor.

**Standardized extract.** An herbal supplement that has been verified to contain a certain percentage of one or more of the herb's active ingredients.

**Stress response.** Series of physiological and biochemical reactions initiated by the hypothalamus when the brain perceives danger or a threat. This is usually a short-lived phenomenon but can become chronic when there are persistent stressors.

**Stroke.** Cerebrovascular accident ("brain attack") in which brain function is lost due to severe disruption of blood and oxygen to the brain.

**Substantia nigra.** Dark-colored area located deep within the cerebrum that is rich in melatonin, the precursor to the neurotransmitter dopamine.

**Synapse.** Gap between two neurons (or between a neuron and an organ) across which nerve impulses are transmitted.

**Temporal lobe.** Portion of the cerebrum that contains the centers for smell and hearing, and some association areas for memory and learning.

**Testosterone.** Steroid hormone that increases male characteristics.

**Thalamus.** Region of the brain that plays a key role in mediating sensation, motor activities, arousal, learning, and memory, and serves as the gateway to the cerebral cortex.

**Thyroid hormones.** Hormones secreted by the thyroid gland that regulate metabolism in every cell of the body. Deficiencies result in depression, lethargy or fatigue, and impaired memory and concentration.

**Trans fatty acid.** Harmful substance produced when vegetable oil is heated and chemically treated to make it solid at room temperature. These fats are linked to heart disease, high cholesterol, diabetes, and cancer.

**Transient ischemic attack (TIA).** Brief episode of cerebrovascular insufficiency caused by partial blockage of an artery to the brain; also called a mini-stroke.

**Tryptophan.** Amino acid that is converted in a two-step process into the neurotransmitter serotonin. Used for its antidepressant and sleep-promoting qualities, tryptophan is available through compounding pharmacies by prescription only.

**Unsaturated fat.** Type of fat found in vegetable oils that has a flexible chemical structure and is liquid at room temperature. *See also* Monounsaturated fat; Polyunsaturated fat.

**Valerian.** Herb that promotes sleep without causing daytime sleepiness or impairment in mental or physical performance.

**Vinpocetine.** Plant-derived nootropic that improves blood flow and oxygen supply to the brain, and protects neurons from the harmful effects of hypoxia. It is used as a therapy for epilepsy, as well as for symptoms of senile dementia and cerebral vascular insufficiency.

**Wernicke's area.** Portion of the brain involved in speech comprehension.

**Working memory.** Also called short-term memory, working memory temporarily holds bits of information from a few seconds to a few hours.

# Resource Section

To obtain most of the vitamins, minerals, essential fatty acids, herbs, amino acids, over-the-counter hormones, and nutrients discussed in this book, check your local health food store. Additional mail-order sources for these and other recommended products are listed below.

Cosmic Sales and Marketing
PO Box 7238
Marietta, GA  30065
800–359–9896
www.newbrain-store.com
www.cris.com/~nubrain
*Source of nootropics and other anti-aging nutrients.*

Healthy Directions, Inc.
Customer Service Center
PO Box 6000
Kearneysville, WV  25430
800–722–8008
www.healthydirections.com
*Source of high-quality nutritional supplements.*

International Antiaging Systems
PO Box 337 - WW
Channel Islands GYI  Great Britain
Phone: 011–44–870–151–4144
Fax: 011–44–870–151–4145
www.antiaging-systems.com
*International source of nootropics.*

Life Enhancement Products, Inc.
PO Box 751390
Petaluma, CA  94975

800–543–3873
www.life-enhancement.com
*Source of vitamins, minerals, nootropics, and other nutrients.*

Masters Marketing Company, Ltd.
Masters House #5,
   Sandridge Close
Harrow, Middlesex, HA1 1TW
England
Phone: 011–44–181–424–9400
Fax: 011–44–181–427–1994
*International source of nootropics.*

Quality Health, Inc. (QHI)
401 Langham House
29–30 Margaret Street
London, W1N 7LB
England
www.qhi.co.uk
*International source of nootropics.*

Vitamin Research Products
3579 Highway 50 East
Carson City, NV  89701
800–VRP–24HR
www.vrp.com
*Source of vitamins, minerals, nootropics, and other nutrients.*

## COMPOUNDING PHARMACIES

For the location of compounding pharmacies in your area, contact the following:

International Academy of
    Compounding Pharmacies (IACP)
PO Box 1365
Sugar Land, TX  77487
800–927–4227
www.iacprx.org

Professional Compounding Centers
    of America (PCCA)
9901 South Wilcrest
Houston, TX  77099
800–331–2498
www.thecompounders.com

## VIDEOS, SOFTWARE, AND BOOKS ON TAPE

Books on Tape, Inc.
PO Box 7900
Newport Beach, CA  92658
800–626–3333
www.booksontape.com
* Provides thousands of unabridged
books on audiotape.

Collage Video
5390 Main Street NE
Minneapolis, MN  55421
800–433–6769
www.collagevideo.com
* Source of over 400 exercise and
workout videos. Free catalog.

Brain.Com
12 Corporate Plaza, Suite 150
Newport Beach, CA  92660
1-888-THINKfast
www.brain.com/thinkfast.htm
* To order THINKfast software.

Nightingale-Conant
7300 North Lehigh Avenue
Niles, IL  60714
800–525–9000
www.nightingale.com
* Provides educational tapes on subjects
ranging from health and political issues
to self-improvement.

## MEDICAL CLINICS

Dr. Stanislaw Burzynski's
    Cancer Institute
12000 Richmond Avenue
Houston, TX  77082
281–597–0111
www.cancermed.com

Whitaker Wellness
    Institute
4321 Birch Street
Newport Beach, CA  92660
949–851–1550
www.whitakerwellness.com

## PHYSICIAN REFERRALS

For a doctor in your area who is knowledgeable in natural hormone replacement, chelation, and other therapies discussed in this book, contact the following:

American Academy of Anti-Aging
  Medicine
1510 West Montana Street
Chicago, IL  60614
773–528–4333
www.worldhealth.net

American College for Advancement
  in Medicine (ACAM)
23121 Verdugo Drive, Suite 204
Laguna Hills, CA  92653
800–532–3688
www.acam.org

Cognitive Enhancement Research
  Institute (CERI)
PO Box 4029
Menlo Park, CA  94026
650–321–2374
www.ceri.com

# References

## Chapter 1 — Memory Loss Is Not Inevitable

Barbour, J. "It's one of life's puzzles: why we remember and why we forget." *Orange County Register,* May 25, 1994.

Cone, W. *Stop Memory Loss: How to Fight Forgetfulness Over 40.* Newport Beach, CA: Matteson Books, 1997.

Costa, PT. Jr., et al. "Psychological research in the Baltimore Longitudinal Study on Aging." *Zeitschrift fur Gerontologie,* 26(3): 138–141, May–June 1993.

Gardner, H. *Frames of Mind: The Theory of Multiple Intelligences.* New York: Basic Books, 1983.

Goleman, D. *Emotional Intelligence.* New York: Bantam Books, 1997.

Schaie, KW. The Seattle Longitudinal Study: a thirty-five-year inquiry of adult intellectual development. *Zeitschrift fur Gerontologie,* 26(3):129–137, May–June 1993.


## Chapter 2 — How Your Brain Works

Benson, H. *Your Maximum Mind.* New York: Times Books, 1987.

Khalsa, DS., and C. Stauth. *Brain Longevity.* New York: Warner Books, 1997.

Lombard, J., and C. Germano. *The Brain Wellness Plan.* New York: Kensington Books, 1997.

Monte, T. *World Medicine.* New York: Jeremy P. Tarcher/Perigee Books, 1993.

Restak, R. *Brainscapes.* New York: Hyperion, 1995.

Sagan, C. *The Dragons of Eden.* New York: Random House, 1977.

Tether, JE. "Brain." *Encyclopedia Americana.* Danbury, CT: Grolier, 1986.

## Chapter 3 — Your Brain at Risk

Baker, B. "NIDDM linked to 30% increased risk of dementia." *Internal Medicine News,* May 15, 1996.

Berg, L., et al. "Clinicopathologic studies in cognitively healthy aging and Alzheimer's disease: relation of histologic markers to dementia severity, age, sex, and apolipoprotein E genotype." *Archives of Neurology,* 55(3):326–335, March 1998.

Bland, JS. "Improving Genetic Expression in the Prevention of the Diseases of Aging." 1999 Seminar Series. Gig Harbor, WA: HealthComm International, 1998.

Bland, JS. "The use of complementary medicine for healthy aging." *Alternative Therapies in Health and Medicine,* 4(4):42–48, July 1998.

Brookmeyer, R., et al. "Projections of Alzheimer's disease in the United States and the public health impact of delaying disease onset." *American Journal of Public Health,* 88(9):1337–1342, September 1998.

Bullido, MJ., et al. "A polymorphism in the regulatory region of APOE associated with risk for Alzheimer's dementia." *Nature Genetics,* 18(1):69–71, January 1998.

Dufouil, C., et al. "Sex differences in the association between alcohol consumption and cognitive performance." EVA Study Group. Epidemiology of Vascular Aging. *American Journal of Epidemiology,* 146(5):405–412, September 1, 1997.

"Faster mental decline in smokers." www.reutershealth.com. April 29, 1998.

Graham, IM., et al. "Plasma homocysteine as a risk factor for vascular disease." The European Concerted Action Project. *Journal of the American Medical Association,* 277(22):1775–1781, June, 11, 1997.

Launer, LJ., et al. "The association between midlife blood pressure levels and late-life cognitive function." The Honolulu-Asia Aging Study. *Journal of the American Medical Association,* 274(23):1846–1851, December 20, 1995.

Lazarou, J., et al. "Incidence of adverse drug reactions in hospitalized patients: a meta-analysis of prospective studies." *Journal of the American Medical Association,* 279(15):1200–1205, April 15, 1998.

Leon, J., et al. "Alzheimer's disease care: costs and potential savings." *Health Affairs,* (Millwood), 17(6):206–216, November–December 1998.

Li, JJ., et al. "Age-dependent accumulation of advanced glycosylation end products in human neurons." *Neurobiology of Aging,* 16(1):69–76, January–February 1995.

Lupien, SJ., et al. "Cortisol levels during human aging predict hippocampal atrophy and memory deficits." *Nature Neuroscience,* 1(1):69–73, May 1998.

McLachlan, DR., et al. "Risk for neuropathologically confirmed Alzheimer's disease and residual aluminum in municipal drinking water employing weighted residential histories." *Neurology*, 46(2):401–405, February 1996.

"Mental decline linked to heart risk factors." www.reutershealth.com. November 9, 1998.

*Physicians' Desk Reference, 1999 (53rd edition).* Montvale, NJ: Medical Economics Data, 1998.

Sacks, O. *The Man Who Mistook His Wife for a Hat.* New York: Summit Books, 1985.

Snowdon, DA., et al. "Brain infarction and the clinical expression of Alzheimer disease." The Nun Study. *Journal of the American Medical Association*, 277(10): 813–817, March 12, 1997.

Strassburger , TL., et al. "Interactive effects of age and hypertension on volumes of brain structures." *Stroke*, 28(7):1410–1417, July 1997.

Werbach, MR. "Does aluminum exposure promote Alzheimer's?" *Nutrition Science News*, 3(1):16–19, January 1998.

## Chapter 4 — Your 10-Step Program

### Step 1   FEED YOUR HEAD

"Are trans fatty acids a serious risk for disease?" Discussion. *American Journal of Clinical Nutrition*, 66(Suppl):1018–1019, 1997.

Blaylock, RL. *Excitotoxins: The Taste That Kills.* Santa Fe, NM: Health Press, 1997.

Fraser, GE., et al. "Variables associated with cognitive function in elderly California Seventh-day Adventists." *American Journal of Epidemiology*, 143(12): 1181–1190, June 15, 1996.

Joseph, JA., et al. "Long-term dietary strawberry, spinach, or vitamin E supplementation retards the onset of age-related neuronal signal-transduction and cognitive behavioral deficits." *Journal of Neuroscience*, 18(19):8047-8055, October 1, 1998.

Schmidt, MA. *Smart Fats.* Berkeley, CA: Frog, Ltd., 1997.

### Step 2   PROTECT YOUR BRAIN WITH VITAMINS AND MINERALS

Benton, D., et al. "The impact of long-term vitamin supplementation on cognitive functioning." *Psychopharmacology (Berlin)*, 117(3):298–305, February 1995.

Benton, D., et al. "Thiamine supplementation, mood and cognitive functioning." *Psychopharmacology (Berlin)*, 129(1):66–71, January 1997.

Chiang, MY., et al. "An essential role for retinoid receptors RARbeta and RXRgamma in long-term potentiation and depression." *Neuron*, 21(6):1353–1361, December 1998.

Clarke, R., et al. "Folate, vitamin $B_{12}$, and serum total homocysteine levels in confirmed Alzheimer disease. *Archives of Neurology,* 55(11):1449–1455, November 1998.

Constantinidis, J. "The hypothesis of zinc deficiency in the pathogenesis of neurofibrillary tangles." *Medical Hypotheses,* 35(4):319–323, August 1991.

Haas, JG. "Study: Vitamin E stalls Alzheimer's." *Orange County Register,* April 24, 1997.

Healton, EB., et al. "Neurologic aspects of cobalamin deficiency." *Medicine,* (Baltimore) 70(4):229–245, July 1991,

Imagawa M., et al. "Coenzyme $Q_{10}$, iron, and vitamin $B_6$ in genetically-confirmed Alzheimer's disease." *Lancet,* 340(8820):671, September 12, 1992.

La Rue, A., et al. "Nutritional status and cognitive functioning in a normally aging sample: a 6-year reassessment." *American Journal of Clinical Nutrition,* 65(1):20–29, January 1997.

Lesser, M. *Nutrition and Vitamin Therapy.* New York: Bantam Books, 1980.

Loriaux, SM., et al. "The effects of nicotinic acid and xanthinol nicotinate on human memory in different categories of age. A double blind study." *Psychopharmacology (Berlin),* 87(4):390–395, 1985.

Meador, K., et al. "Preliminary findings of high-dose thiamine in dementia of Alzheimer's type." *Journal of Geriatric Psychiatry and Neurology,* 6(4):222–229, October–December 1993.

Murray, M., and J. Pizzorno. *Encyclopedia of Natural Medicine.* Rocklin, CA: Prima Publishing, 1998.

Pelton, R., and T. Pelton. *Mind Food and Smart Pills.* New York: Doubleday, 1989.

Pyapali, GK., et al. "Prenatal dietary choline supplementation decreases the threshold for induction of long-term potentiation in young adult rats." *Journal of Neurophysiology,* 79(4):1,790–1,796, April 1998.

Riggs, KM., et al. "Relations of vitamin B-12, vitamin B-6, folate, and homocysteine to cognitive performance in the Normative Aging Study." *American Journal of Clinical Nutrition,* 63(3):306–314, March 1996.

Rosenberg, IH., and JW Miller. "Nutritional factors in physical and cognitive functions of elderly people." *American Journal of Clinical Nutrition,* 55 (6Suppl):1237–1243, June 1992.

Sano, M., et al. "A controlled trial of selegiline, alpha-tocopherol, or both as treatment for Alzheimer's disease." The Alzheimer's Disease Cooperative Study. *New England Journal of Medicine,* 336(17):1216–1222, April 24, 1997.

Schmidt, R., et al. "Plasma antioxidants and cognitive performance in middle-aged and older adults: results of the Austrian Stroke Prevention Study." *Journal of the American Geriatric Society,* 46(11):1407–1410, November 1998.

Shevell, MI., and DS Rosenblatt. "The neurology of cobalamin." *Canadian Journal of Neurological Science,* 19(4):472–486, November 1992.

Sinatra, ST. *The Coenzyme $Q_{10}$ Phenomenon.* New Canaan, CT: Keats Publishing, 1998.

Subar, AF., et al. "Fruit and vegetable intake in the United States: The baseline survey of the Five a Day for Better Health Program." *American Journal of Health Promotion,* 9(5):352–360, May–June 1995.

Tucker, DM., et al. "Nutrition status and brain function in aging." *American Journal of Clinical Nutrition,* 52(1):93–102, July 1990.

van Goor, L., et al. "Review: cobalamin deficiency and mental impairment in elderly people." *Age and Aging,* 24(6):536–542, November 1995.

"Vitamin A aids memory, learning." www.reutershealth.com. January 8, 1999.

## Step 3  RESTORE MEMORY WITH HERBS

Allain, H., et al. "Effect of two doses of ginkgo biloba extract (EGb 761) on the dual-coding test in elderly subjects." *Clinical Therapeutics,* 15(3):549–558, May–June 1993.

Kleijnen, J., and P. Knipschild. "Ginkgo biloba." *Lancet,* 340(8828):1136–1139, November 7, 1992.

Le Bars, PL., et al. "A placebo-controlled, double-blind, randomized trial of an extract of Ginkgo biloba for dementia." North American EGb Study Group. *Journal of the American Medical Association,* 278(16):1327–1332, October 22–29, 1997.

Murray, MT. *The Healing Power of Herbs.* Rocklin, CA: Prima Publishing, 1995.

Oken, BS., et al. "The efficacy of Ginkgo biloba on cognitive function in Alzheimer disease." *Archives of Neurology,* 55(11):1409–1415, November 1998.

## Step 4  NURTURE YOUR BRAIN WITH FATS

Crook, TH., et al. "Effects of phosphatidylserine in age-associated memory impairment." *Neurology,* 41(5):644–649, May 1991.

Crook, TH., and B. Adderly. *The Memory Cure.* New York: Pocket Books, 1998.

Kidd, PM. "Phosphatidylserine; membrane nutrient for memory. A clinical and mechanistic assessment." *Alternative Medicine Review,* 1(2):70–84, April 1996.

Schmidt, MA. *Smart Fats.* Berkeley, CA: Frog, Ltd., 1997.

Soderberg, M., et al. "Fatty acid composition of brain phospholipids in aging and in Alzheimer's disease." *Lipids,* 26(6):421–425, June 1991.

Willatts, P., et al. "Effect of long-chain polyunsaturated fatty acids in infant formula on problem solving at 10 months of age." *Lancet,* 352(9129):688–691, August 29, 1998.

## Step 5 Exercise for Peak Mental Performance

Dustman, RE., et al. "Aerobic exercise training and improved neuropsychological function of older individuals." *Neurobiology of Aging,* 5(1):35–42, Spring 1984.

Goldman, R., et al. *Brain Fitness.* New York: Doubleday, 1999.

Khalsa, DS., and C. Stauth. *Brain Longevity.* New York: Warner Books, 1997.

Steinberg, H., et al. "Exercise enhances creativity independently of mood." *British Journal of Sports Medicine,* 31(1):240–251, September 1997.

## Step 6 Sharpen Your Mind With Mental Workouts

Allen, ADW. "Glycemically Acceptable/Unacceptable Foods." www.anndeweesallen.com/dal_gly.htm.

"Brain cells can regenerate." www.reutershealth.com. October 30, 1998.

Carughi, A., et al. "Effect of environmental enrichment during nutritional rehabilitation on body growth, blood parameters and cerebral cortical development of rats." *Journal of Nutrition,* 119(12):2005–2016, December 1989.

Crook, TH., and B. Adderly. *The Memory Cure.* New York: Pocket Books, 1998.

Diamond, MC., et al. "Plasticity in the 904-day-old male rat cerebral cortex." *Experimental Neurology,* 87(2):309–317, February 1985.

Eriksson, PS., et al. "Neurogenesis in the adult human hippocampus." *Nature Medicine,* 4(11):1313–1317, November 1998.

Franklin, D. "Playing games." *Hippocrates,* 67–71, December 1997.

Hollander, J. *Committed to Memory.* New York: Books & Co./Turtle Point, 1996.

Khalsa, DS., and C. Stauth. *Brain Longevity.* New York: Warner Books, 1997.

McCraty, R., et al. "The effects of different types of music on mood, tension, and mental clarity." *Alternative Therapies in Health and Medicine,* 4(1):75–84, January 1998.

Michaud, E., and R. Wild. *Boost Your Brain Power.* Emmaus, PA: Rodale Press, 1991.

Miller, JB., et al. *The G.I. Factor: The Glycemic Index Solution.* Sydney, Australia: Hodder Headline, 1996.

Nudo, RJ., et al. "Use-dependent alterations of movement representations in primary motor cortex of adult squirrel monkeys." *Journal of Neuroscience,* 16(2):785–807, January 15, 1996.

Rauscher, FH., et al. "Music and spatial task performance." *Nature,* 365 (6447):611, October 14, 1993.

Rideout, BE., and CM Laubach. "EEG correlates of enhanced spatial performance following exposure to music." *Perceptual and Motor Skills,* 82(2):427–432, April 1996.

Sarnthein, J., et al. "Persistent patterns of brain activity: an EEG coherence study of the positive effect of music on spatial-temporal reasoning." *Neurological Research,* 19(2):107–116, April 1997.

Schaie, KW. The Seattle Longitudinal Study: a thirty-five-year inquiry of adult intellectual development. *Zeitschrift fur Gerontologie,* 26(3):129–137, May–June 1993.

Schmidt, MA. *Smart Fats.* Berkeley, CA: Frog, Ltd., 1997.

Snowdon, DA., et al. "Linguistic ability in early life and cognitive function and Alzheimer's disease in late life. Findings from the Nun Study." *Journal of the American Medical Association,* 275(5):528–532, February 21, 1996.

Xerri, C., et al. "Plasticity of primary somatosensory cortex paralleling sensori-motor skill recovery from stroke in adult monkeys." *Journal of Neurophysiology,* 79(4):2119–2148, April 1998.

**Step 7  REDUCE MIND-NUMBING STRESS**

Casa Marasco, A., et al. "Double-blind study of a multivitamin complex supplemented with ginseng extract." *Drugs under Experimental and Clinical Research,* 22(6):323–329, 1996.

D'Angelo, L., et al. "A double-blind, placebo-controlled clinical study on the effect of a standardized ginseng extract on psychomotor performance in healthy volunteers." *Journal of Ethnopharmacology,* 16(1):15–22, April–May 1986.

de Quervain, DJ., et al. "Stress and glucocorticoids impair retrieval of long-term spatial memory." *Nature,* 394(6695): 787–790, August 20, 1998.

Hallstrom, C., et al. "Effect of ginseng on the performance of nurses on night duty." *Comparative Medicine East and West,* 6:277–282, 1982.

Holmes, TH., and RH Rahe. "The social readjustment scale." *Journal of Psychosomatic Research,* 11:213–218, August 1967.

Kinzler, E., et al. "Effect of a special kava extract in patients with anxiety, tension, and excitation states of non-psychotic genesis. Double blind study with placebos over 4 weeks." *Arzneimittel-Forschung,* 41(6):584–588, June 1991.

Linde, K., et al. "St John's wort for depression—an overview and meta-analysis of randomized clinical trials." *British Medical Journal,* 313(7052):253–258, August 3, 1996.

Lupien, SJ., et al. "Cortisol levels during human aging predict hippocampal atrophy and memory deficits." *Nature Neuroscience,* 1(1):69–73, May 1998.

"Prolonged cortisol elevation linked to memory deficit in elderly." www.reutershealth.com. April 15, 1998.

Regelson, W., and C. Colman. *The Superhormone Promise.* New York: Simon & Schuster, 1996.

"Siberian ginseng (Eleutherococcus senticosus): current status as an adapto-gen." *Economic and Medicinal Plant Research,* eds. H. Wagner, Hiroshi Hikino, and Norman R. Farnsworth, 1:156–215, 1985.

## Step 8   REJUVENATE YOUR BRAIN WITH SLEEP

Aldrich, MS., and JE Shipley. "Alcohol use and periodic limb movements of sleep." *Alcoholism, Clinical and Experimental Research,* 17(1):192–196, February 1993.

Arendt, J., et al. "Alleviation of jet lag by melatonin: preliminary results of controlled double blind trial." *British Medical Journal,* Clinical Research Edition, 3; 292(6529):1170, May 1986.

Coren, S. *Sleep Thieves.* New York: The Free Press, 1996.

Dawson, D., and K. Reid. "Fatigue, alcohol and performance impairment." *Nature,* 388(6639):235, July 17, 1997.

Dressing, H., et al. "Insomnia: are Valeriana/Melissa combinations of equal value to benzodiazepine?" *Therapiewoche,* 42:726–736, 1992.

Johnson, S. "Inside TMI: Minute by Minute." www.wowpage.com/tmi.

King, AC., et al. "Moderate-intensity exercise and self-rated quality of sleep in older adults. A randomized controlled trial." *Journal of the American Medical Association,* 277(1):32–37, January 1, 1997.

Kleitman, N. *Sleep and Wakefulness.* Chicago: University of Chicago Press, 1963.

Phillips, BA., and FJ Danner. "Cigarette smoking and sleep disturbance." *Archives of Internal Medicine,* 155(7):734–737, April 10, 1995.

"Power naps keep workers alert." www.reutershealth.com. March 18, 1997.

"Sleep deprivation common, says survey." www.reutershealth.com. March 25, 1998.

"Sleep deprivation lowers percentage of natural killer cells in blood." www.reutershealth.com. June 15, 1997.

"Sleep deprivation while driving called a major public health threat." www.reutershealth.com. May 29, 1996.

Wolfe, SM, and R. Hope. *Worst Pills Best Pills II.* Washington, DC: Public Citizen's Health Research Group, 1993.

## Step 9   ENHANCE BRAIN FUNCTION WITH HORMONES

"Androderm Testosterone Transdermal System." U.S. Prescribing Information. SmithKline Beecham, 1997.

Barnes, BO., and L. Galton. *Hypothyroidism: The Unsuspected Illness.* New York: Harper-Collins, 1976.

Birge, SJ. "The role of estrogen in the treatment of Alzheimer's disease." *Neurology,* 48(5 Suppl 7):S36–41, May 1997.

Flood, JF., et al. "Memory-enhancing effects in male mice of pregnenolone and steroids metabolically derived from it." *Proceedings of the National Academy of Sciences of the United States of America,* 89(5):1567–1571, March 1, 1992.

Guth, L., et al. "Key role for pregnenolone in combination therapy that promotes recovery after spinal cord injury." *Proceedings of the National Academy of Sciences of the United States of America,* 91(25):12,308–12,312, December 6, 1994.

Jacobs, DM., et al. "Cognitive function in nondemented older women who took estrogen after menopause." *Neurology,* 50(2):368–373, February 1998.

Kawas, C., et al. "A prospective study of estrogen replacement therapy and the risk of developing Alzheimer's disease: the Baltimore Longitudinal Study of Aging." *Neurology,* 48(6):1517–1521, June 1997.

Murphy, DD., and M. Segal. "Regulation of dendritic spine density in cultured rat hippocampal neurons by steroid hormones." *Journal of Neuroscience,* 16(13):4059–4068, July 1, 1996.

Pincus, G., et al. "Effects of administered pregnenolone on fatiguing psychomotor performance." *Aviation Medicine,* 98–135, April 1944.

Regelson, W., and C. Colman. *The Superhormone Promise.* New York: Simon & Schuster, 1996.

Resnick, SM., et al. "Estrogen replacement therapy and longitudinal decline in visual memory. A possible protective effect?" *Neurology,* 49(6):1491–1497, December 1997.

Sunderland, T., et al. "Reduced plasma dehydroepiandrosterone concentrations in Alzheimer's disease." *Lancet,* 2(8662):570, September 2, 1989.

"Testosterone supplements may improve memory in older men." www.reutershealth.com. July 7, 1998.

Wolkowitz, OM., et al. "Dehydroepiandrosterone (DHEA) treatment of depression." *Biological Psychiatry,* 41(3):311–318, February 1, 1997.

Wright, JV., and L. Lenard. *Maximize Your Vitality and Potency.* Petaluma, CA: Smart Publications, 1999.

**Step 10** STRENGTHEN MEMORY WITH SMART DRUGS AND NUTRIENTS

Alvarez, XA., et al. "Citicoline improves memory performance in elderly subjects." *Methods and Findings in Experimental and Clinical Pharmacology,* 19(3):201–210, April 1997.

Calatayud Maldonado, V., et al. "Effects of CDP-choline on the recovery of patients with head injury." *Journal of the Neurological Sciences,* 103 (Suppl): S15–18, July 1991.

Cipolli, C., and G. Chiari. "Effects of L-acetylcarnitine on mental deterioration in the aged: initial results." *Clinica Terapeutica*, 132(6 Suppl):479–510, March 31, 1990.

Croisile, B., et al. "Long-term and high-dose piracetam treatment of Alzheimer's disease." *Neurology*, 43(2):301–305, February 1993.

Dimpfel, W., et al. "Source density analysis of functional topographical EEG: monitoring of cognitive drug action." *European Journal of Medical Research*, 1(6):283–290, March 19, 1996.

Dow, A. *Deprenyl: The Anti-Aging Drug.* Clearwater, FL: Hallberg, 1993.

Dutov, AA., et al. "Use of cavinton in epilepsy." *Zhurnal Nevropatologii I Psikhiatrii Imeni S. S. Korsakova*, 86(6):850–855, 1986.

Hindmarch, I., et al. "Efficacy and tolerance of vinpocetine in ambulant patients suffering from mild to moderate organic psychosyndromes." *International Clinical Psychopharmacoly*, 6(1):31–43, Spring 1991.

Hindmarch, I., et al. "The effects of an ergot alkaloid derivative (Hydergine) on aspects of psychomotor performance, arousal, and cognitive processing ability." *Journal of Clinical Pharmacology*, 19(11–12):726–732, November–December 1979.

Lawson, WE., et al. "Efficacy of enhanced external counterpulsation in the treatment of angina pectoris. *American Journal of Cardiology*, 70(9):859–862, October 1, 1992.

Levin, HS. "Treatment of postconcussional symptoms with CDP-choline." *Journal of the Neurological Sciences*, 103 (Suppl):S39–42, July 1991.

Lino, A., et al. "Psycho-functional changes in attention and learning under the action of L-acetylcarnitine in 17 young subjects. A pilot study of its use in mental deterioration." *Clinica Terapeutica*, 140(6):569–573, June 1992.

Lozano Fernandez, R. "Efficacy and safety of oral CDP-choline. Drug surveillance study in 2817 cases." *Arzneimittel-Forschung*, 33(7A):1073–1080, 1983.

Mindus P., et al. "Piracetam-induced improvement of mental performance. A controlled study on normally aging individuals." *Acta Psychiatrica Scandinavica*, 54(2):150–160, August 1976.

Pfeiffer, CC., et al. "Stimulant effect of 2-dimethyl-l-aminoethanol: possible precursor of brain acetylcholine." *Science*, 126:610–611, 1957.

Olszewer, E., and JP Carter. "EDTA chelation therapy in chronic degenerative disease." *Medical Hypotheses*, 27(1):41–49, September 1988.

Sacks, O. *Awakenings.* New York: Summit Books, 1985.

Schmidt, U., et al. "Piracetam in elderly motorists." *Pharmacopsychiatry*, 24(4):121–126, July 1991.

Schneider, LS., and JT Olin. "Overview of clinical trials of hydergine in dementia." *Archives of Neurology*, 51(8):787–798, August 1994.

Skolnick, AA. "Old Chinese herbal medicine used for fever yields possible new Alzheimer disease therapy." *Journal of the American Medical Association,* 277(10):776, March 12, 1997.

Smith, BH., and J. Dreyfus. *The Broad Range of Clinical Use of Phenytoin.* New York: Dreyfus Medical Foundation, 1992.

Spagnoli, A., et al. "Long-term acetyl-L-carnitine treatment in Alzheimer's disease." *Neurology,* 41(11):1726–1732, November 1991.

Spiers, PA., et al. "Citicoline improves verbal memory in aging." *Archives of Neurology,* 53(5):441–448, May 1996.

Subhan, Z., and I. Hindmarch. "Psychopharmacological effects of vinpocetine in normal healthy volunteers." *European Journal of Clinical Pharmacology,* 28(5):567–571, 1985.

Xu, SS., et al. "Efficacy of tablet Huperzine-A on memory, cognition, and behavior in Alzheimer's disease." *Chung Kuo Yao Li Hsuch Pao,* 16(5):391–395, September 1995.

# Index

# Whitaker Wellness Institute
# Medical Clinic

Since 1979, the Whitaker Wellness Institute Medical Clinic in Newport Beach, California, has attracted thousands of people who suffer from a variety of medical concerns, including failing memory and cognitive function, heart disease, diabetes, high blood pressure, high cholesterol, hormone imbalance, prostate conditions, irritable bowel syndrome, osteoporosis, asthma and allergies, thyroid conditions, weight problems, and autoimmune disorders. Through the clinic's unique one-week Back to Health Program, staff physicians safely guide patients to improved health through the integration of nutritional supplementation, specialized alternative therapies, conventional treatments, diet, and exercise.

For additional information about the clinic:
1–800–488–1500
www.whitakerwellness.com.

# *Health & Healing* Newsletter

*Health & Healing,* Dr. Julian Whitaker's monthly newsletter, is nationally recognized as a leading source of alternative health information. In each issue, Dr. Whitaker presents the latest research on proven complementary treatments, as well as step-by-step guidelines on how to use vitamins, minerals, herbs, and other natural therapies effectively for improved health. Subscribers also receive a copy of the comprehensive Whitaker Wellness Program for good health.

For additional information about *Health and Healing:*
1–800–539–8219
www.DrWhitaker.com

# Healthy Habits

*are easy to come by—*

## IF YOU KNOW WHERE TO LOOK!

### Get the latest information on:
- **better health • diet & weight loss**
- **the latest nutritional supplements**
- **herbal healing • homeopathy and more**

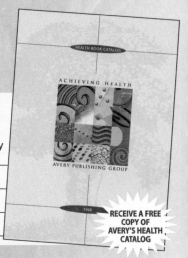

RECEIVE A FREE
COPY OF
AVERY'S HEALTH
CATALOG

## COMPLETE AND RETURN THIS CARD RIGHT AWAY!

**Where did you purchase this book?**
- ❏ bookstore
- ❏ health food store
- ❏ pharmacy
- ❏ supermarket
- ❏ other (please specify)_____

Name_____

Street Address_____

City_____ State_____ Zip_____

---

## GIVE ONE TO A FRIEND ...

# Healthy Habits

*are easy to come by—*

## IF YOU KNOW WHERE TO LOOK!

### Get the latest information on:
- **better health • diet & weight loss**
- **the latest nutritional supplements**
- **herbal healing • homeopathy and more**

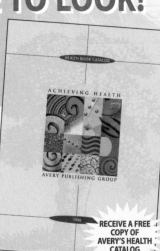

RECEIVE A FREE
COPY OF
AVERY'S HEALTH
CATALOG

## COMPLETE AND RETURN THIS CARD RIGHT AWAY!

**Where did you purchase this book?**
- ❏ bookstore
- ❏ health food store
- ❏ pharmacy
- ❏ supermarket
- ❏ other (please specify)_____

Name_____

Street Address_____

City_____ State_____ Zip_____

## Avery Publishing Group

**120 Old Broadway**
**Garden City Park, NY 11040**

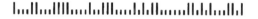

## Avery Publishing Group

**120 Old Broadway**
**Garden City Park, NY 11040**